Mindful Alignment

Mindfulness in Education

Series Editors: Karen Ragoonaden and Sabre Cherkowski, The University of British Columbia

This interdisciplinary series examines the theoretical and the practical applications of Mindfulness in Education (MIE). Coming from a range of academic disciplines, an increasing number of studies on mindfulness and related contemplative practices underscore the relevance of MIE. Prompted by the robust scientific findings of mindfulness as a tool to support physical, emotional, and mental health in adult populations, several initiatives have emerged devoted to applying and evaluating mindfulness in K–12 and in higher education. Teachers are enrolling in mindfulness programs, administrators are introducing mindfulness to their schools, and researchers are devising ways to evaluate the effects of mindfulness in cohorts of students and teachers. In particular, the collected volumes of this series explore the impact of universal practices of mindfulness (being aware, paying attention, noticing, being in the present moment, being nonjudgmental) and the attributes that cultivate and support well-being in pedagogical contexts.

Titles in the Series

Mindful Alignment

Foundations of Educator Flourishing

Sabre Cherkowski,
Kelly Hanson,
and
Keith Walker

LEXINGTON BOOKS
Lanham • Boulder • New York • London

Published by Lexington Books
An imprint of The Rowman & Littlefield Publishing Group, Inc.
4501 Forbes Boulevard, Suite 200, Lanham, Maryland 20706
www.rowman.com

Unit A, Whitacre Mews, 26-34 Stannary Street, London SE11 4AB

British Library Cataloguing in Publication Information Available

Library of Congress Cataloging-in-Publication Data

Names: Cherkowski, Sabre, 1970- author. | Hanson, Kelly, 1979- author. | Walker, Keith D. (Keith Douglas), 1954- author.
Title: Mindful alignment : foundations of educator flourishing / Sabre Cherkowski, Kelly Hanson, and Keith Walker.
Description: Lanham : Lexington Books, [2018] | Series: Mindfulness in education | Includes bibliographical references and index.
Identifiers: LCCN 2018006170 (print) | LCCN 2018003909 (ebook) | ISBN 9781498570794 (Electronic) | ISBN 9781498570800 (pbk. : alk. paper) | ISBN 9781498570787 (cloth : alk. paper)
Subjects: LCSH: Reflective teaching. | Mindfulness (Psychology)
Classification: LCC LB1025.3 (print) | LCC LB1025.3 .C453 2018 (ebook) | DDC 371.102--dc23
LC record available at https://lccn.loc.gov/2018006170

Contents

Introduction

*Toward Crafting Architectures to Nurture
the Educator's Soul*

What does it mean to flourish as an educator? This simple question about what it means to pay attention to wellbeing and to learn to thrive as an educator has been at the heart of our research on flourishing in schools, and serves as the centering question for this book on mindful alignment. There is no *right* answer to the question, just as there is no *right* way to thrive as an educator. When we learn to pay attention to wellbeing, our own and others', as a central aspect of our work and our vocation, we are generating a contextualized understanding of what we need to be at our best. We believe that awareness of wellbeing is foundational for flourishing in the work of teaching, learning, leading, and living well together, through, and in, the role of educator. While simple in its statement, the pursuit of flourishing, in the many different ways it may be assumed and experienced, is a complex challenge for educators.

Over the last several years we have engaged in research with teachers and other school leaders to learn about how they sense flourishing in their work. We have aimed to learn about how we can start noticing and growing wellbeing in schools from the perspective of educators, so that they can flourish in their work and model and promote wellbeing in their students and others in the learning community (c.f. Cherkowski & Walker, in press; 2014; 2016). Through this research, we have found that the process of structuring educators' work in ways that promote flourishing for self and others in learning communities is easier said than done; however, attending to this complex issue is essential. We need to start paying attention to wellbeing for the sake of our educator colleagues, our students, our families, and our communities.

We need those who lead the learning and development of our children and youth to feel well, whole, and alive in their work in order to best meet the demands faced by us, and to meet the needs of our young people, now and in the future. We cannot afford to walk away from this challenge, nor will our passive indifference produce the flourishing we want for others, and for ourselves. We recognize the enormity of this task within the current challenges facing many educators who experience stress, exhaustion, and burnout due to increasing demands placed on already overextended work lives. Within this reality, we do strongly call for more focus on wellbeing at a systemic level—supporting and encouraging teacher wellbeing is not something that should be left only to individuals to sort out, build up, or sustain. Educator wellbeing requires system-level attention and resources. As researchers and teacher educators, we count ourselves as part of the process for attending to wellbeing as an organizational issue, and continue to research, write, and teach for change in schools, so that wellbeing is at the forefront of how we organize schools.

Of course, we should not wait for systems to change when we know that there are practices, strategies, and ways of thinking, doing, knowing, and being that provide adjustments or slight tweaks toward greater wellbeing for individual and groups of educators. We see this as part of a systemic approach to reorienting school organizations toward flourishing. We need to provide information and encouragement for individual educators, on their own and within groups, to attend to their self-care as central to their work of teaching and learning in schools. As authors, we aim to provide information and insight to teachers that encourage them to pay attention to small adjustments within their own domains of action toward what we call "mindful alignments." We share how these alignments make a world of positive difference in educators' journeys toward flourishing.

We believe this journey toward educators learning to flourish in their work is meaningfully experienced as a communal one, and we invite you to join with us as we explore the ways practicing mindful awareness provides a new space for opening and expanding our minds, hearts, and bodies, as we attend to what make us feel whole, alive, and well in our work and life. We know that each person's journey of flourishing can, and often does, look quite different than the next person's. Moreover, supporting flourishing needs to happen in ways that honor the notion that the movement toward flourishing is an ongoing aspiration rather than a fixed endpoint. We see this shift in perspective toward an intentional focus on flourishing at work—in the many different ways that it will be experienced—as an integral part of reclaiming the importance of wellbeing for educators.

From our research with educators about what it means to flourish, from the research of others in various fields, and from our own experiences as educators aiming for more wellbeing in our work and lives, we have conceptualized a model of mindful alignment that highlights three central aspects toward which we can focus our attention:

- our wellbeing
- our relationships
- our unique passions and strengths

Mindful awareness of these three aspects provides a focus for how our values, beliefs, and goals align with our actions, responses, intentions, and desires for crafting and expressing our best selves in and through the work of teaching. We see the work of developing mindful alignment as a process of professional learning for flourishing, and suggest that this can be facilitated through a series of practices, or arts of mindful alignment. We call the mindful practices for mindful alignment "arts," after Langer (2005), who describes artistry as an ongoing process of learning about the world through self-discovery, and art as a capacity that we can all mindfully cultivate through the *doing* of art. This professional learning process of paying attention, and then practicing the arts of mindful alignment to grow our capacities in each of the three aspects—wellbeing, relationships, strengths and passions—is a kind of mindful awareness and is foundational for flourishing.

SHIFTING TOWARD A POSITIVE, APPRECIATIVE, AND GENERATIVE PERSPECTIVE

Our research reflects our interest in bringing to education findings from the growing research fields of positive psychology and positive organizational studies that focus on the positive and generative aspects of life and work, such as happiness, joy, flow, delight, among other positive emotions and states. For example, we now understand that a focus on positive emotions in one aspect of life can contribute to increasing capacities and capabilities in other areas of our lives (Fredrickson, 2008). Research in positive organizations has demonstrated that achieving a level of positivity in the workplace can be generative, life-giving, and beneficial across many levels of the workplace. As an example of a positive state that teachers might experience toward their own sense of flourishing, we have considered Mikhaly Csikszentmihaly's (1997) research on the construct of "flow." Flow is a psychological state of joy produced from engagement in an activity in which individuals demonstrate an intense and focused concentration, a sense of losing track of time, a loss of self-consciousness, a feeling of control of one's actions and environment, and high levels of intrinsic satisfaction (Csikszentmihalyi, 1997; Nakamura & Csikszentmihalyi, 2014; Seligman, 2011). We encourage educators to pay attention to how these positive attributes and capacities may

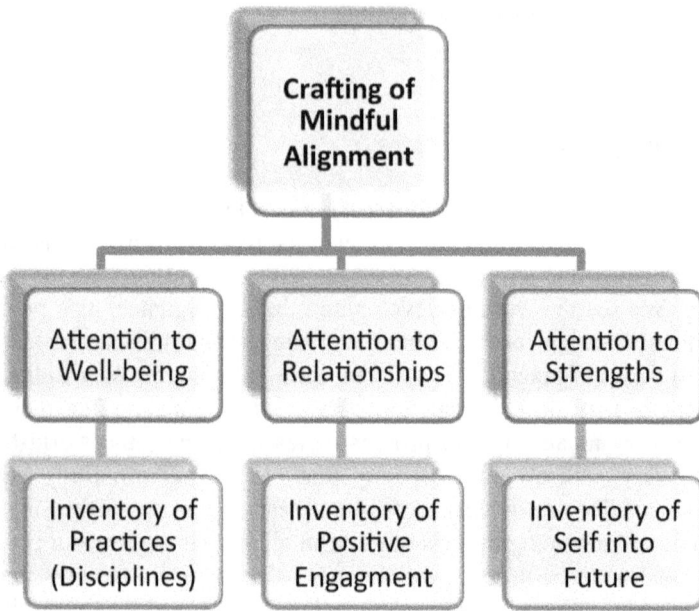

**Figure 0.1.   Crafting Mindful Alignment: Paying Attention and Practicing Arts.
Figure created by authors.**

be cultivated in the work of teaching, leading, and learning in schools because each holds the promise and potential for positive improvement in many
aspects of school life. Thich Nhat Hanh (2017) describes *happy teachers as
those who will change the world.* He offers that mindfulness practices help
bring awareness to the mind and body, and that over time educators can use
this awareness to "reduce tension and develop confidence, clarity, compassion, ease, and joy" (Hanh, 2017, xxvi). Mindfulness, according to Hanh, is a
path to experiencing less suffering. His perspective very much aligns with
our own positive approach to human development by taking human strengths
as a starting point for building what is possible. This perspective does not
deny suffering or suggest that there are quick fixes, but rather suggests that
cultivating what is good is possible, and to cultivate good creates more
flourishing.

MINDFUL ALIGNMENT:
A PRACTICE FOR GROWING WELLBEING

One of the ideas we promote is that wellbeing can be understood as a complex phenomenon, experienced differently by different people, and one that

includes many facets, such as our inherent agency to determine a certain level of wellbeing through our mindful awareness of our selves and those around us. We know that there are many aspects of life beyond our control and that these sometimes throw a big wrench into our plans to attain and sustain wellbeing. For example, we know through Larry Crabb (1990) and Stephen Covey (1989) that a person can and should only take responsibility for those things within their control. Our goals need to be focused on what we can do, and on what no one else can block or interfere with. For example, our agency allows us to determine our values and goals, and enables us to see how our goals (inside our realm of influence and control) differ from our desires, dreams, and concerns, which often exceed what we can directly influence or control. By paying attention to this difference, we focus on what we can do and avoid a great deal of frustration, anger, or worry about that which is beyond our personal and professional sovereignty (i.e., other people, institutions, or circumstances). Nonetheless, there are "effects" that may result from our being, doing, and daring inside our operational sphere that are out of our control. While we don't have the power to stop these troublesome wrenches or disruptions, we have seen through our own and others' research that humans have a unique capacity for pausing, reflecting, and choosing a response to almost any situation we face, finding resilience in whatever circumstances might be thrown at us. Pause and reflection are integral to establishing the parameters for responses that reflect our values, goals, desires, intentions, and influences, so that we are then able to choose to respond in ways that align with what works in aid of our flourishing. We call this mindful awareness process "mindful alignment," and suggest that it is an ongoing, lifelong, and life-wide learning journey that can bring us closer toward a realization of flourishing in our life and work.

Much like our original question about wellbeing, we know that the suggestion to pay attention to how we, ourselves, hold the agency for determining our own wellbeing may seem simplistic, rosy, and overly optimistic. However, we hope to demonstrate that this path of self-knowing, self-reflection, and self-cultivation is a complex and challenging life path that holds immeasurable benefits and rewards for us and for those we care for. As indicated, we will explore spaces for practicing mindful alignment through attending to wellbeing, relationships, and our own passions and strengths as central to the work of educators. Through an ongoing practice of mindful awareness with attention on alignment of our responses, attitudes, beliefs, and actions, we can craft, over time, selves that reflect our values, passions, and purpose. As we will show, this crafting does not happen in isolation, but through the many relationships that form the social worlds within which we work and live.

PAYING ATTENTION TO WHOLENESS THROUGH ARTS OF MINDFUL ALIGNMENT

When we say that we need to pay attention to growing wellbeing for ourselves and others as the work of teaching, we mean that humans are wonderfully complex, with minds, hearts, and bodies, and that wellbeing comprises all these aspects of who we are. We have built a fairly broad conceptualization of what it means to be a flourishing educator—beyond merely teaching practices, duties, responsibilities, and tasks—to focus on the wholeness of the person who is the educator, to shine a light on the fullness of the human. We aim to bring attention to what we call the "hidden architecture of the educator's soul." As we conceptualize it, at the center of the architecture of the educator's soul there is the unique and precious human spirit, with capacities of mind, emotions, and a sense of agency. Parker Palmer (1999a) suggests, "If we are to open up the spiritual dimension of education, we must understand that spiritual questions do not have answers in the way math problems do—and that giving one another The Answer is part of what shuts us down. When people ask these deep questions, they do not want to be saved but simply to be heard: they do not want fixes or formulas but compassion and companionship on the demanding journey called life" (p. 8). We agree with Palmer that these questions can prompt deeper thinking and feeling about what it means to live our lives as educators, and that the act of asking the question engages us in an inquiry into the spiritual dimensions of our work-lives at school. Our intention through this book is to offer learning opportunities for paying attention to these often hidden questions in ourselves through engaging in mindful awareness of our wellbeing, of the relationships in our work and life, and of how we express our unique passions and strengths. This learning process can lead us to craft mindful alignment toward revealing the hidden architecture of our educator souls, one that reflects our authentic and flourishing selves.

One focus of this mindfulness is related to our purpose and our identity, becoming aware of who we are and why we exist through noticing the stories that we, with others, construct about our social world. This attention to story as a path toward making meaning in our work represents our engagement, awareness of flourishing moments, our sense of self-efficacy (what we can do to learn and grow), and eventually the experience of patterns of flourishing (where our mindful practices and crafting is habituated). In addition to purpose and identity, we think that a person's passions and strengths are a key element to the architecture of their soul. As we seek to be consistent with our true self (the person we are called to be), we recognize our unique passions and strengths and then build on these to make room for ourselves to be authentic persons of integrity. Of course, our purpose and identity are connected to our passions and our strengths. Our awareness of, and attunement to, these dimensions of our lives are important. We are also persons of promise and agency. We have two things in mind in our use of the word "promise":

- We are persons of potential, capacities, and capabilities—we hold promise for transcendence, to become better today than yesterday and better tomorrow than today. We are growing into, and transforming through, our learning into the most promising person we might be.
- We are persons who are more than self-referent; we are agentic. We are bound in relationship to others. There is an exchange and, in so many ways, we are the beneficiaries of others, reciprocating the generosity of others' contributions to our lives, in our promise or agreement to serve others.

As professionals, we act on behalf of the best interests of others and the higher and common good. We live and serve in environments of relational grace (Palmer, 2004). We have natural, psychological and legal obligations as persons to other persons—we are social beings who exchange in synergistic, symbiotic, serendipitous, and synchronistic fashions with others in the exercise of our promise.

As we connect our purpose and identity, our passions and strengths, and our promise and agency through personal practices and professional crafting, we engage in the work and play of making our occasional moments of flourishing more frequent and qualitatively enriched. We begin to experience more flow, fruitfulness, joy, and fulfillment. We become more fit, happy, and well. So again, the focus of this book is on how mindful alignment, with attention to three aspects—wellbeing, relationships, and our unique passions and strengths—through practicing mindful arts and crafting can assist educators to flourish, with the hope that they will then influence, promote, and encourage others to embark on their own learning journey toward flourishing.

CRAFTING A SELF THROUGH MINDFUL AWARENESS

Crafting opportunities for self-awareness and uncovering the architecture of the soul of the flourishing educator are metaphors that resonate with our assumptions about the social construction of reality, our beliefs about the human capacity for agency, creativity, and building a life of meaning and purpose. We hope these design metaphors will call out to the wholeness of who you are—that these will beckon a sense of tuning in to your most precious and wondrous self as we prompt you to reflect on your mind, body, and spirit in and through your work in education. This architecture and agency for building our best self is present in each of us. We hope to provide the prompts and calls that help to bring these metaphors to greater awareness. We also offer examples of how greater awareness of self and design agency can be lived out in our work through practices such as job crafting. In our own situations we have experienced job crafting, where we have used our awareness of our wellbeing to establish or shift structures in our work to promote or sustain our sense of wellbeing. For example, we have collaborated with colleagues in (re)structuring our teaching days with students to share courses and classes in ways that build on our unique areas of passion and strengths. We have also experienced smaller crafting moments of shifting around, when and where we can, the various responsibilities in our day, such as email, to the afternoon to make room for larger blocks of uninterrupted time for creative works, such as writing. We hope that your engagement with the ideas in this book will prompt you to explore, expand, and enjoy the architecture of your own flourishing and design ways to scaffold and strengthen this architecture in your work context. There is agency in developing this level of self-awareness; an opportunity to keep what is working well for you and to shed what is not.

Uncovering the hidden architecture of the soul of a flourishing educator sounds like serious work, and so it is. However, we think this serious work is best taken up in playful and joyful ways. It is a learning journey into what makes us feel most alive, engaged, in tune, and in touch with ourselves and with others with whom we work and live. This is a joyous journey, and it is also a quest. Joseph Campbell is most well known for his writing on the connections between the myths that we culturally tell and our human consciousness. Campbell (1949) is also known for his description of the "hero's journey." The hero's journey is a process that begins when an individual accepts the call to become the greatest version of him- or herself. From there, the journey is long and winding, with many trials and tribulations. Campbell describes the "dark night of the soul" as an individual's time of difficult contemplation and time of suffering. We see that the call to flourishing is a quest that requires courage to question beliefs and practices, especially neutral or dysfunctional ones. While the hero's journey may be carried out in solitude, we see the flourishing quest as best undertaken in community, and, when possible, with a light and open heart. Through this book, we offer you our companionship in your journey. We offer the theory and practices im this book as a modest lighthouse to guide you on your quest, and to hopefully inspire you to join with other educators to make sense of the spirited nature of this work.

Through our research with educators, we have learned the importance of companionship at work. Companionship is often nurtured through opportunities to share food. How interesting that the tender and simple acts of community, such as dining together, can create the space for the mindful work that can help answer the call to the greatest self within the context of community. As we frame our work within a mindfulness perspective, we notice that this creates a sense of wholeness (mind, emotions, volition, body, and spirit), of abundance and of fulfillment. Often the work of the teacher is approached from a purely cognitive perspective, and we see that this approach sometimes misses the other important aspects of who we are. Using an eclectic blend of theories, research findings, reflections, and practices that notice and nurture an alignment of mind, body, and spirit, we aim to bring to awareness the hidden architecture of the soul of flourishing educators. We invite you to join with us on a learning journey toward deeper and greater understanding of self as the renewed starting point on your quest toward sustaining a life of flourishing.

INVITING YOU TO NOTICE YOUR CALLING, YOUR AGENCY, AND YOUR ASPIRATION TO FLOURISH

We have found that the language we use to describe our reality is a powerful tool for creation. The idea that we can access our thoughts and harness them in ways that move us forward toward a desired future is powerful and has been researched from a variety of theoretical perspectives. For example, in psychology, logo-therapy highlights the importance of harnessing the power of an individual to search for the meaning in each experience by noticing the ways we can link or craft our response to any given experience to align with our core values, or the intentions we have for how we aim to live. Framing our response toward a choice that aligns our actions with our values can create opportunities for building meaning out of every situation. Through the exercise of this choice for meaning, we create our freedom in any situation (Frankl, 1959; 1984; Pattakos, 2010).

Acceptance and commitment therapy (ACT) is a more recent psychological theory that builds on the idea that humans have a unique capacity to choose their responses to any given situation by attending, in a mindful way, to the realities of the present. This is done in such a way that we face the present as it currently is, not as we wish it would be, and then choose a response that aligns with our desires for who we hope to be in the future (Harris, 2009). Through practicing mindful awareness in our lives, and learning to choose responses and actions that align with our deepest values, we can start to improve the quality of our experiences.

From organizational research literature we also see this theme of the potential and power inherent in the ways we verbalize or express our social realities. From an open, appreciative, and mindful perspective, our language enables us to engage in action in ways that move us forward in constructing an image of the future that most inspires us toward a higher version of ourselves. For example, appreciative inquiry is an approach to organizational change that builds from the idea that language and thoughts are powerful forces for creating an image of a desired future such that individuals and groups are motivated to work together to attain that vision (Cooperrider & Shrivasta, 1987). The appreciative inquiry approach to positive change is predicated on social constructionist principles that argue that the language we use to describe our social realities creates those realities as we talk about them. In other words, how we talk about our work and life makes us feel certain ways and influences how we behave. Aligned with this assumption, learning to attend to how we use language to story our lives is an important aspect of developing an architecture of the soul that aligns with our values, intentions, and desires for who we are and how we engage with others through our work and life.

Through our research, we have found that appreciative perspectives provide opportunities for educators to learn to pay attention in new and generative ways to the questions they ask, the stories they tell, and the lens they use to view their work. These have potential for profound improvement in our work and our lives. However, shifting toward engaging in our worlds with a flourishing lens requires ongoing practice for many of us. In this work we have noticed a relationship between improving mindful awareness and growing flourishing. As we focus our awareness on that which gives us life, breathes life, nurtures life, then we become more fully alive. We have found that paying attention to these processes, as part of the work of professional learning, has traction with educators and provides momentum and impetus for engaging in the work of mindful alignment.

This book is an invitation to learn about what it means to you to flourish as an educator. This is a personal learning journey about coming to know yourself, learning what matters to you, asking what makes you come alive at work, and learning about the highest versions of yourself that are offered in the service of encouraging those around you to join in on their own personal journey of learning about flourishing. This is an invitation and it is also a call. It is a call for an expanded understanding of professional development to include the deep learning necessary to come to an awareness of self in relation to others and to the worlds that we are continually creating with each other. It is a call for organizing schools in ways that encourages ongoing learning about what it means to flourish as human beings in educator roles. This call has been at the heart of our research for several years, as we have sought to learn from educators about what it means to them to flourish at work, and to learn about how they attend to their ongoing self-growth, learning about and then living out at work their best selves, when they more often feel nudged and needled to respond to so many competing demands that can leave them feeling stressed out and depleted. As we have engaged with educators, we better understand the value and importance of wellbeing as central to the work of teaching and learning. We have learned the importance of paying attention to building quality relationships at work, and we recognized the need for educators to become empowered to notice and live out a higher purpose in their work. These ideas provide a theoretical umbrella for the practices that we will offer throughout this book for cultivating mindful awareness.

A START TO YOUR OWN LEARNING JOURNEY: ORGANIZATION OF THE BOOK

Through this book we share our assumptions about the possibilities for shifting the way we think about the work of teaching, learning, and leading in schools toward one that foregrounds notions and theories of appreciation, abundance, strength, and virtue orientations, and human development approaches to how we organize and work within schools. We provide our insights and understandings about what it means to flourish in school. Throughout the book, we have woven theory and practice for flourishing, using research from studies in positive psychology and positive organizations, mindfulness, and professional learning, with practices that we have collected from our research participants and their efforts to create space for reimagining human flourishing in schools, as well as from practices collected from mindfulness and other self-care domains. Each chapter is a blend of theory and practice ending with suggested arts for mindful alignment.

We offer these examples as a starting point for you to begin your own inquiry into what makes you come most alive, feel connected and engaged in your work. As we have sought to learn ways to leverage what others have described as working well and offer these as clues for how to keep growing in new places and new ways, we invite you to take what you learn here and use these insights to leverage your own shift in perspective toward flourishing. Our foundational beliefs are that everyone can flourish, and that flourishing is a unique and recursive process of mindful alignment. We have described flourishing as connected to an awareness of the human spirit at work, and we aim to explore more deeply the practices that develop our attention and create the flourishing moments in our lives.

In chapter 1, we offer a description of mindfulness as a method for developing the mind's capabilities through awareness of the mind, a way to live in harmony with oneself and in touch with others (Kabat-Zinn, 1994). In chapter 2, we start our description of the mindful alignment model with attention to wellbeing through the mindful art of attuning to disciplines of abstinence and engagement as a way of noticing how we are living out our aspirations for wellbeing in our daily lives. In chapter 3, we highlight the second aspect of mindful alignment, the importance of building relationships in professional cultures, and we describe attuning to the body and the mindful art of listening. In chapter 4, we describe the importance of paying attention to purpose and higher meaning as the third aspect of mindful alignment through the art of attuning to personal strengths and values. In chapter 5, we offer our suggestions for attuning to the mindful design of our work through the art of job crafting. We conclude with chapter 6, mindful awareness as a foundation for flourishing, wherein we return to our premise for shifting our perspective toward flourishing, and the value of using an appreciative, generative, social constructionist view of our social realities.

Chapter One

Mindfulness and Mindful Alignment

A Lifelong Professional Learning Process

We developed the term *mindful alignment* after reading MacDonald and Shirley's (2009) writing on teaching inquiry into mindful teaching, and how this inquiry served to build a growing awareness of how mindfulness perspectives and practices provide new opportunities for professional learning. Exploring what it means to engage as a mindful teacher, through a series of ongoing workshops and conversations with teachers, MacDonald and Shirley (2009) highlight authentic alignment as one of seven pillars or practices of mindful teaching. They suggest that authentic alignment of teachers' personal and professional ethics with their actions is at the core of what it means to have a sense of fulfillment and engagement as a teacher. They acknowledge the complexity of mindful teaching, and the challenges of balancing contemplation with action. Mindful teaching is about coming to know when we are in or out of authentic alignment, and about being able to take steps toward recalibrating our work, and ourselves, toward a sense of alignment.

These tensions and challenges facing educators who aim to engage more mindfully in their work were also shared with us by the teachers in our research project. Teachers shared the challenges of balancing professional workloads that seemed to endlessly encroach on their personal and family time. They struggled to balance the desire to work on behalf of improving the educational experiences of their students with their desires to have full and meaningful personal lives. They struggled to balance their desires to advocate for their students with their desires to support and advocate for their colleagues or, more broadly, for their school organization. Through our work with them, we offered a new way to think about their struggles. Recognizing and acknowledging these very real challenges, we asked them to reflect in a different way, and to use different practices, such as appreciative reflections, to access understandings, experiences, and moments in their work where they felt alive, engaged, and whole as educators, and then to notice what happened in their work as they focused on these arts of their practice.

We have found that alignment for flourishing happens over and over again as one appreciates what it means to fully engage in the work of teaching. This alignment requires courage and compassion for self and others. Teaching happens as part of a professional collective where educators work toward engaging and enriching their students' lives. This can raise tensions for educators who belong to a collective of professionals while, at the same time, maintaining their authentic alignment and agentic selfhood. We suggest that learning to grow our knowledge of self is an essential aspect of moving into community, enabling us to engage with curiosity, compassion, and courage to work with others in a more open, present, and authentic way of being (Cherkowski, Hanson, & Kelly, 2014). We see that mindful alignment develops through ongoing professional learning that supports the development of attention to wellbeing, positive relationships, and strengths, passions, and purposes. Over time, this deep sense of alignment that emerges from ongoing practice of mindful awareness of self becomes a foundation for flourishing, our own and others'.

To create a context and provide the theories about mindfulness that underpin our mindful alignment model, we offer an overview of mindfulness from two complimentary but separate perspectives. The first is from a psychological perspective that focuses on cognitive awareness of mindsets and learning patterns as a way of understanding the difference between mindlessness, and mindfulness. Second, we describe a mindful inquiry stance that informs for us what it can mean to engage as a mindful teacher. From these theories and experiences, we describe processes and practices that are helpful for engaging in developing mindful alignment. Finally, we further develop our conceptualization of mindful alignment as coming into awareness of who we are, what we value and believe, and how this is enacted in relation in our various contexts.

THE IDEA OF MINDFULNESS

The idea of mindfulness is increasingly indicated as an important practice in personal and professional development. There is growing interest about how to use mindfulness to decrease stress and increase positive traits and habits for the quality of our lives. From a psychological perspective, mindfulness may be understood as "the awareness that emerges through paying attention on purpose . . . to the unfolding of experience moment by moment" (Kabat-Zinn, 2003, p. 14), through contemplative techniques and practices, such as meditation. Research results confirm that as teachers have adopted mindfulness programs and practices for their classrooms that there have been positive behavioral and emotional results. These include enhanced memory, an increased ability to concentrate, an effective means to regulate emotions, and an increased expression of empathy and compassion (Greenberg et al., 2003; Jennings & Greenberg, 2009; Meikeljohn et al., 2012; Schonert-Reichl & Lawlor, 2010). These studies connect the science of how the brain changes through an ongoing practice of meditation techniques with a focus on social-emotional learning.

Mindfulness has been described as being fully aware in the present moment through contemplative connections of mind, body, and spirit (Rodgers & Raider-Roth, 2006; Newmark, Krahnke, & Seaton, 2013). This synergy between mental, emotional, and physical states is said to enable individuals to make thoughtful decisions from a perspective of clarity that comes from being present. This mindfulness perspective can also contribute to persons taking more risks in their learning and making discoveries about themselves, rather than their merely making automatic decisions based on previous experience (Rodgers & Raider-Roth, 2006). In other words, if a person's complete attention is focused and present, they are able to be fully aware of their emotions and they are able to control and concentrate on the tasks at hand (Newmark et al., 2013). When a person makes a conscious effort to live in the present moment, there are benefits experienced in terms of emotional self-regulation and flexibility within situations that afford good decisions. This, in turn, leads to further success in life (Meiklejohn et al., 2012). This kind of mindfulness moves practitioners beyond their thoughts and allows them to connect with their hearts and spirits in everyday life and circumstances.

Techniques such as meditation, body scans, and mindful walking are often used to engage in the practice of purposefully paying attention without judgment to the present moment. While many of these practices originated in Buddhist traditions, they have been combined with other traditional practices and adapted for use in Western medicine, social work, nursing, education, business, and other sectors. Based on growing neuro-scientific research showing the plasticity of the brain and the ability for the brain to continue to grow and develop through important for personal and professional development. There are certainly mental benefits from meditation, such as improved attention, focus, memory, creativity, and other cognitive abilities. Mindfulness has been shown to provide benefit for our wellbeing during the actual practice and, as a residual effect of the practice, throughout the remainder of the day. This wellbeing is experienced at the physical level, as our brain and body benefit from hormone surges that are released as we enter into states of deep relaxation (Seigel, 2007).

Paying attention to the breath, through meditation, mindful walking, yoga, and other practices, is often the suggested anchor for beginning and maintaining a state of mindful awareness. Paying attention to the breath, and to the body as the breath moves through it, is an effective cue for learning to grow attention. As thoughts move through our minds, as they will, the goal is to not attach to them, but rather to let them pass through while we attend to the breath. In this way, we can learn to see that thoughts come and go and that we have an ability to attend to them or not, attach to them or not, ascribe meaning to them or not (Brown & Olson, 2015; Marturano, 2014). Through ongoing practice we can learn to notice and let go of unnecessary thoughts as they arise, even when not in meditation. Through meditation, the brain develops new pathways that are less reactive to stress, anger, and frustration, and these pathways provide us the space to pause, notice, and then determine how we wish to act on stressful or negative thoughts or situations. This is in contrast to reacting automatically with the well-worn brain pathways from anger, frustration, and other inflammatory responses. Mindfulness can provide the space in our minds for allowing us to respond to stressors from a more thoughtful, creative, and caring way that alleviates anger, frustration that can lead to stress and then burnout (Davidson et al., 2003; 2013). Over time with ongoing training, some of the benefits of a regular mindfulness practice include improved abilities to: notice and slow down automatic reactions, see more clearly and respond more adaptively to complex situations, and achieve a greater sense of balance, resilience, and compassion (Brown & Olson, 2015; Marturano, 2014). Meditation provides the training to cultivate space between our experience and our reactions, and allows us to choose more pro-social responses such as kindness, connection, and humor. Mindfulness practices also boost our abilities to cultivate compassion and kindness.

MINDFULNESS IN EDUCATION

Given that the research findings from medicine and psychology indicate that physical, mental and emotional benefits occur with regular mindfulness practice, secular adaptations of mindfulness activities such as breath practices, meditation, and yoga are making an increasing impact in classroom practices and in teacher development. In an overview of research on classroom-based mindfulness training for students and teachers, Meikeljohn et al. (2012) describes findings across fourteen studies where mindfulness practices for students and teachers decreased anxiety and stress, and improved attention, memory, and other academic and social skills as well as improving overall emotional regulation.

Mindfulness-based programs for teachers are typically designed to reduce stress and improve resilience. Research has found positive outcomes of these programs, such as improved capacities to respond to the stress of the work of teaching in productive, healthy, and compassionate ways (Flook et al., 2013; Jennings et al., 2013). Through these programs, teachers learn meditation practices that focus attention on the breath and mental scans of the body to notice tension, pain, and unease, as well as reflective exercises to reframe experiences in more emotionally healthy ways. Continued research is necessary to learn more about how to best support educators in developing mindfulness practices in order to alleviate the effects of stress and anxiety that seem so widespread in teaching and to provide a more openhearted approach to the work of teaching (Roeser et al., 2012).

From a cognitive learning perspective, mindfulness may be understood as an excellent means for engaging with our perceptions of the world in a curious, flexible, and open-minded way. Ellen Langer's (1997) ideas of mindfulness presume several psychological states, such as: "1) openness to novelty; 2) alertness to distinction; 3) sensitivity to different contexts; 4) implicit if not explicit awareness of multiple perspectives; and 5) orientation to the present" (p. 23). From her research, Langer describes how most of us are habituated in our routines and ways of seeing the world so that much of what we do happens on automatic pilot, mindlessly. Engaging from a mindful approach to anything requires what she calls "sideways learning," to stay open to novelty and multiple possible experiences. For teachers, mindful teaching encourages students to question and wonder about other potential ways of engaging with the material or finding answers in a variety of ways. This is a more conditional view of learning that offers students the opportunity to engage more meaningfully in understanding content, gaining skills, and developing capacities from a more personal and individually relevant way. Langer (1989) also addresses the psychological and physical costs of mindlessness and how the practice of mindfulness can lead to a sense of control, greater freedom of action and possibilities, and less burnout. Fortified by research, Langer explains how and why mindlessness develops and then shows how we can become more mindful and oriented in the present.

THE NATURE OF MINDLESSNESS

Mindlessness is restrictive by nature. Mindlessness may be described as being entrapped by categories, as predictably leading to educators under- or overreacting to situations with automatic behaviors and acting from a single standpoint or from an inflexible perspective. Mindlessness occurs as we blindly and rigidly adhere to categories, ideations, inferences, and distinctions created in the past. These categories tend to lock us into an identity,

with rules and responses for particular actions and with prescribed interpretations of how and why things happen as they do. For example, as people
engage in group think and other behaviors, they may do so without actively
and consciously paying attention to the details or nuances. This may result in
what we could call mindless activity. Langer (1989) asserts, "When we
blindly follow routines or unwittingly carry out senseless orders, we are
acting like automatons, with potentially grave consequences for ourselves
and others" (p. 4). Mindlessness develops as we engage in repeated behaviors
over a period of time, resulting in the formation of habits. Mindlessness also
manifests itself when people operate as though there were only one set of
rules, one perspective, or a single way to interpret a situation, so that other
options are excluded. Langer (1989) describes such behavior: "Our minds
snap shut like a clam on ice and do not let in new signals" (p. 18). All three
elements—entrapment by categories, automatic behavior, and acting from a
single perspective—work against mindfulness and may be seen as mindlessness.

THE CAUSES OF MINDLESSNESS

Langer (1989) maintains that the elements of repetition, premature cognitive
commitment, belief in limited resources, the notion of linear time, education
for outcome, and ignoring the vital role of context have direct impact on the
roots of mindlessness. Repeating a task to learn to perform it without thought
can lead to mindlessness. Langer (1989) writes that "[a] familiar structure or
rhythm helps lead to mental laziness, acting as a signal that there is no need
to pay attention" (p. 21). A second cause of mindlessness is termed "premature cognitive commitment," whereby one accepts and commits to an "im-
pression or a piece of information at face value, with no reason to think
critically about it" (p. 22). When singular mindsets are formed in childhood,
rigid commitment often deters the possibility of considering other options or
viewpoints at a later time. Langer (1989) states: "The way we first take in
information (that is, mindfully or mindlessly) determines how we will use it
later" (p. 25). Third, beliefs in limited resources lead to entrenched mindlessness. Langer (1989) asserts, "If there are clear and stable categories, then we
can make rules by which to dole out these resources" (p. 27). For example, it
was once believed that humans could not run the mile in fewer than five
minutes. However, the record has been broken and the supposed limit extended. As another example, Langer gives the case of a divorcing couple
with a child. Rather than the resource-restricted question, "Who gets the
child?" she suggests that consideration should be given to the complexity of
what is actually being sought. Langer writes that, "A child's love is not a
zero-sum commodity. Two people can love and be loved by a child. Feelings

are not a limited resource" (p. 28). It is when people perceive that the necessary things in life are in short supply that rigid categories are clung to and are "mindlessly entrapping us" (Langer, 1989, 29). In fact, many of the limits we accept as real are illusory, because people can do more than they originally thought possible.

Langer's fourth criteria of mindlessness is the linear view of time that restricts possibilities and contributes to mindlessness. Langer (1989) describes other cultures and people groups who view time as a universal present, as cyclical, or as a means of organizing perception. Linear time is likened to a closed system, where people imagine they have a sense of control. A fifth element that contributes to mindlessness is how early education emphasizes predetermined outcomes and goals as opposed to the process by which they are achieved. A preoccupation with outcomes can make us singularly minded on achieving success and avoiding failure, rather than concentrating on our natural desire to explore and to be curious. The child is focused on "Can I do it?" rather than on the mindful question of "How do I do it?" Langer (1989) writes that, "The style of education that concentrates on outcomes generally also presents facts unconditionally. This approach encourages mindlessness. If something is presented as an accepted truth, alternative ways of thinking do not even come up for consideration" (p. 35). According to Langer, the sixth element that contributes to mindless thinking is the way that context contributes to behavior. Langer uses the illustration that a roller coaster ride is fun, but that bumpy plane rides are not. Many of the contexts that deeply affect an individual are those we learned in childhood and have become a mindset. We assume that others will behave in the same manner, in the same context, and when it is otherwise, it is termed context-confusion. These six elements—repetition, premature cognitive commitment, belief in limited resources, the notion of linear time, education for outcome, and the role of context—are various causes of mindlessness and influence how one engages in the world.

THE RESULTS OF MINDLESSNESS

Langer (1989) discusses five detrimental results of mindlessness: an inhibited self-image, unintended cruelty, limited options, loss of control, and stunted potential. First, when educators define themselves according to a narrow role, purpose, or image, they may become vulnerable when the situation or the rules change. For example, when an educator has narrowly defined herself as a grade two teacher and mother of three children and discounts her roles as daughter, sister, friend, and artist, she may feel a loss of identity if she moves to teach grade five and her children grow up and move away. Of course, "grade two teacher" and "mother of three school-aged children" are wonderful designations, just not sufficient to tell the whole story.

We can also feel that our self-image is threatened when mindlessly comparing ourselves to others, when the focus is placed on outcomes rather than on the process or effort others put into becoming successful. Langer (1989) asserts that, "When we envy other people's assets, accomplishments, or characteristics, it is often because we are making a *faulty comparison*. We may be looking at the *results* of their efforts rather than at the *process* they went through on the way" (p. 46). Rather, it is important to identify the process or the steps anyone must take to be successful. In addition, a self-image based on past performance may also be threatening to one's sense of identity. For example, a lack of success experienced in the past does not mean the same for the future; rather, we can learn that putting in the needed effort, training, and determination leads to success. Negative mindsets that are established in the past may inhibit improvement and growth. Also, if we accept negative labels for our selves, even though we may be capable of learning or performing a skill, performance and learning will be undermined. Thus, mindlessness may contribute to a negative self-image. Mindlessness may also cause insensitivity and unintended cruelty to others. Perceiving others who are different or who have disabilities often results from mindless assumptions, resulting in discrimination or prejudice. By not questioning our behavior, by falling into a routine, or by disregarding the life experiences of others, "we can get mindlessly seduced into activities we wouldn't engage in otherwise," says Langer (1989, p. 49).

Langer also describes how mindlessness can limit our control by preventing intelligent choices. For example, when advertisers make statements that seduce shoppers, they often do so with the notion that little thinking goes into the purchase. As people perceive that certain troubles are attributed to a single cause, options become limited and people may give up their sense of control. Learned helplessness can occur as we experience a sense of futility and a loss of control and choice. Repeated failure or submissive resignation to situations may lead to mindlessness and loss of our determination and perseverance. Langer (1989) writes that, "Even when solutions are available, a mindless sense of futility prevents a person from reconsidering the situation" (p. 54). Because of a loss of hope, no effort is put forward to make a way through. Furthermore, our potential may be stunted due to premature cognitive commitments. Langer is particularly interested in how negative perspectives of aging that were formed in childhood by caregivers turn out to influence not only patient care but also the self-image of the aging person. If the aged are perceived as incompetent and senile, then their actions may be viewed through those lenses.

In summary, mindlessness diminishes our self-image, narrows choices, ties us to single-minded attitudes, and minimizes our contributions to a life of thriving. We provide next a description of the alternative mindset, mindfulness.

THE NATURE OF MINDFULNESS

"Our life is what our thoughts make it." —Marcus Aurelius, *Meditations*

In contrast with mindlessness, mindfulness is characterized by continually creating new categories, by welcoming new information, by attending to more than one perspective, by increasing a sense of control, and by focusing on process rather than outcome. First, mindful persons adapt to their environment by categorizing and recategorizing, or labeling and relabeling, as opposed to rigidly and mindlessly adhering to old categories. We form new categories in a mindful way by attending to the particular elements of a situation and to its context. As an educator extends beyond global categories and is mindful of new distinctions and differentiated categories, engrained and apparently limiting opinions can change. For example, our negative attitude toward a person, situation, or object may change as we look for more detail, information, explanations, or possibilities.

Second, a mindful state implies that the educator is open to new information, cues, and changes in the environment. Langer (1989) advocates that "behaviour generated from mindful listening or watching, from an expanding, increasingly differentiated information base" (p. 67). It is important to keep an open mind and to operate from a continuous feedback loop.

Third, Langer (1989) advocates that openness, not only to new information, but also to different points of view, is a mark of mindfulness. To be aware of other viewpoints, interpretations, and perspectives will help to build understanding and strengthen social interactions. Langer (1989) writes that "every idea, person, or object is potentially simultaneously many things depending on the perspective from which it is viewed. A steer is steak to a rancher, a sacred object to a Hindu, and a collection of genes and proteins to a molecular biologist" (p. 69). As we consider different perspectives, choices, empathy, and change become more possible.

A fourth benefit of practicing mindfulness is that it better enables the educator to change mental contexts. In a study where patients were given a more optimistic context to think about while in hospital (i.e., playing football or preparing for a dinner party of ten), they could better control their experience of pain. Mindfulness is characterized by focusing on something new and fascinating. Boredom is a construct of the mind and works against mindfulness. A fifth element of mindfulness is its orientation toward the process rather than the outcome. Intentional choices are made for mindful reasons. As mindful persons work toward particular outcomes, they go through important processes that may include learning through trial and error, practicing perseverance, and redoing and recategorizing. If an educator is focused only on outcome, then their self-esteem may be threatened through paying attention to accomplishments of others without giving due regard to the work or process they, themselves, are engaged in. Langer (1989) says, "A process orientation not only sharpens our judgment, it makes us feel better about ourselves. A purely outcome orientation can take the joy out of life" (p. 76).

As we have indicated, the nature of mindfulness includes the elements of continually creating new categories, of welcoming new information, of attending to more than one perspective, of increasing a sense of control, and of focusing on process rather than outcome.

MINDFUL PROFESSIONAL LEARNING

For educators, mindful professional learning encourages ongoing questioning of our assumptions, routines, and practices, and promotes our inquiring into novel ways to engage our students and ourselves to learn to be responsive to the present and sensitive to the diversity of contexts that shape and influence us all. For example, the text *A Mindful Teaching Community* (Hanson, 2017) is a collection of stories from a group of educators who developed a collective mindful practice in order to study and improve their teaching practices. Over time, the educators attributed their strengthened sense of connection to each other to group meditation and contemplation practices. It seemed that mindfulness shifted and improved how they collaborated with each other and led to exciting revelations about creativity, pursuits of justice, and ecological awareness. Hanson writes that "through mindful practice, we learned to value and understand each other's gifts and perspectives. I think mindfulness can offer this to us all. As a global teaching community, we can share a commitment to shift, grow, and change by learning from each other though kindness, love, and compassion" (2017, p. xii).

We suggest that all educators could gain a deeper understanding of ourselves in relation to others through their own practices of mindful inquiry. Over time, this can become their own path toward personalized professional learning. We hope to support such inquiry by describing how becoming aware of how our actions resonate with our beliefs and values opens new possibilities for the flourishing educator self. When we feel most alive, engaged, and authentic, we are flourishing. Mindful alignment entails becoming attuned to the discrepancy between our acting self and our intentioned self, using continuous learning about ourselves and others in our work and in life in general. As we tune up our self-awareness, self-acceptance, and self-care, we gain authenticity on the path toward experiencing flourishing. We suggest that cultivating and nurturing mindful alignment is an essential aspect of ongoing professional learning, a process of mindful inquiry.

MINDFUL INQUIRY

As an educator, you are in an intellectual profession that requires constant inquiry into your practice. Teaching is a highly complex phenomenon that cannot be improved by simply following how-to lists or procedures handed down by someone outside of your practice context (Darling-Hammond, 2010; Zeichner, 2010). It requires you to carefully plan and carry out your actions to nurture students' wholistic development (Inoue, 2015, p. 2).

There are different conceptions of mindful inquiry presented across social scientific research. Leading this work is the seminal text *Mindful Inquiry in Social Research* by Bentz and Shapiro (1998). The authors of this text describe mindful inquiry as an approach to research that not only makes space for, but focuses on the creative, contextual, and personal aspects of the researcher as the primary concern of the research. The philosophy behind Bentz and Shapiro's mindful inquiry combines four intellectual traditions: Buddhism, critical theory, hermeneutics, and phenomenology. We suggest that learning more about the intellectual traditions described by Bentz and Shapiro as the cornerstone philosophies of mindful inquiry (1998, p. 67) is worthwhile. Ongoing meditation on these theories by teachers, in light of their practices, could help them generate new knowledge about the world around them. For our discussion, we focus on the scholar-practitioner nature, or sense-making nature, of mindful inquiry, also emphasized by Bentz and Shapiro, in light of theories of wellbeing such as flourishing. A scholar-practitioner is an educator who draws on theory and practice in order to inquire into their experiences and to make sense of them in order to improve student learning. It is a practice of continual questioning. Mindfulness practices and associated practices of awareness such as deep listening, nonjudgment, and appreciation improve the quality of our noticing, and, in turn, our questions can shift and change. We are hopeful that our readers will draw on the theories of wellbeing offered throughout this book to make sense of their practices in ways that help them grow their own flourishing.

Engaging in mindful inquiry means we need to learn to examine the beliefs, assumptions, and worldviews that inform and guide our actions, and to recognize that these are social and historical in nature. Time, space, and place matter when it comes to how we internalize and live out our worldviews. Mindful inquiry is the process of coming to know one's self in relation to others, and in relation to the life-worlds that we navigate in our human journeys. Coming to know who we are in relation to our social worlds is the very process of an authentic learning journey toward mindful alignment, as we attune to our best selves in the service of encouraging all others to do the same.

Engaging with colleagues in cycles of inquiry aimed toward improving student outcomes is an established and widely accepted method for school improvement. This is evidenced by the increasing popularity of professional learning community initiatives and teacher inquiry groups in schools. Indeed, our own and others' research on collaborative, inquiry-based professional development for teachers highlights the promise for meaningful change in schools when teachers are encouraged and supported to engage with their colleagues in continuous cycles of reflection on their practices (Cherkowski & Schnellert, 2017; Samaras, 2011; Schnellert & Butler, 2014; Cochran-Smith & Lytle, 2009). Mindful inquiry extends and enriches collaborative teacher inquiry practices by turning the gaze inward, toward a reflective awareness of one's self, as the starting point for inquiry with colleagues (Ragoonaden & Bullock, 2016). As Inoue (2015) describes it, mindful inquiry starts with an examination of beliefs and assumptions.

One of the greatest challenges of being a human being is attuning to our perceptions, since the seemingly natural ways we navigate relationships, interpret the world, and present ourselves are often invisible to us. We take our perceptions for granted, we make assumptions, and easily find ourselves in autopilot mode. Ellen Langer describes the danger of these automated ways—not only the physical dangers of not being aware (the limited reflexes and delayed response time from our conditioned states), but also the loss of meaning experienced because of the missed opportunities to deepen our ways of thinking and being through noticing multiple perspectives. When we are operating from autopilot mode, we have shut down or ignored the opportunity to learn and grow from multiple perceptions and perspectives in ways that open us up to the possibilities of experiencing novel and unique understandings and interpretations of our social and natural worlds.

For the purposes of this book, we define mindfulness as an intentional, appreciative state of mind that seeks out, acknowledges, and assumes multiple perspectives. This mindfulness is experienced as an openness to novelty and learning (Inoue, 2015; Langer, 1989; 1993) about ourselves, others, and the worlds in which we work and live. What we have noticed through our research is that the insight gained from a mindful perspective, from noticing what is happening in our own minds, hearts, and bodies through our constructed perception is a worthwhile and transformative practice. Inoue (2015) explains that a hallmark of the Western tradition of thinking is the desire to "overcome uncertainty and ambiguity" (p. 7). Through mindful inquiry, educators learn to become more comfortable with the uncertainty that is inherent in all learning, and to pay attention to how this uncertainty may become the opportunity to align their displayed behaviors and attitudes with their intended beliefs and actions.

MINDFUL ALIGNMENT: A LIFELONG PROFESSIONAL LEARNING JOURNEY

We are educators of educators. We teach in university teacher education programs, working with those who aspire to be teachers, and with school teachers who come back to graduate school to enhance their professional understandings and skills for their work. We know about the importance of reflection in the work of education. In our early careers as classroom teachers, we were socialised into the processes of regularly reflecting on what we do with our students and then determining whether or not what we did led to the outcomes we had hoped. In this way, we learned to shift our activities to achieve the desired outcomes. Constant calibration is a way of life for the educator. This ongoing reflection is part of what it means to be a good teacher, and has been emphasized as both a personal and a collective activity necessary for moving toward improving student learning. We have spent many years of research and teaching about how to best improve schools through enhanced educator professional development. We know this enhancement of professional development for improving student learning can happen through engagement in professional learning communities designed for classroom-, school-, and district-level changes. Reflection in these communities is fostered through staff members inquiring together, regularly and rigorously reflecting on practices that influence student learning, and determining whether or not these practices are pedagogically and organizationally strong and responsive.

More recently, we have shifted our own inquiry and reflections on professional development toward new ways of thinking and seeing the work of teaching, leading, and learning in schools. We have been wondering what happens if we shift our questions to notice what gives us life in our work, what provokes vitality and zest, what makes us feel aware, engaged, motivated, enthused, curious, and invested. We have wondered what would happen if we explicitly noticed professional development for school improvement using more appreciative and compassionate lenses. We noticed that shifting the lenses that we used to ask our questions has provided an opening for new ways of understanding what it means to organize schools for the work of teaching, learning, and leading. Over the past several years, we have been engaged in research designed to elicit an understanding of what works well in teachers' work lives, so as to contribute to building a research base of positive organizational knowledge and practices of flourishing across many schools. We have written about these findings in several articles and book chapters (Cherkowski & Walker, 2014; 2015; 2016; 2017), providing our interpretations—guided by our theoretical framework of the stories shared to us by our participants—about how to shift the way we organize and work within schools toward a focus on what works well and makes us feel engaged and energized. We engaged in this research with a mindful attention to how we, as researchers, were reflecting on, attending to, and shifting toward habits and capacities of flourishing in our own work as a research team, with our graduate research assistants, and within and through the relationships we were building with our school sites and with participants.

We share here a brief overview of our research methodology that resonates with ideas and assumptions about what it means to engage in mindful inquiry. In our case, we were researching what it means for teachers to feel a sense of flourishing in their work. We designed a set of principles and practices that we came to understand as a Flourishing Inquiry methodology that is more fully described in our other writing (Cherkowski & Walker, 2017). We provide here a snapshot of this methodology to describe or highlight how we engaged in the research that formed the underpinnings for conceptualizing mindful alignment for flourishing.

Early in the research process, we established a set of research principles from which we would work together as a team (including graduate research assistants and participants) that aligned with the principles and values of the theoretical framework that underpinned the research (positive organizational scholarship, positive psychology, learning community theory and research). These principles became the foundational pillars of the research and were intended to serve as a reminder to design and engage in the research in ways that encouraged further flourishing. In other words, we saw this research as an opportunity to be a catalyst to grow wellbeing through the processes that we would design to work with participants in schools. We also saw this as an opportunity to grow our own wellbeing through this work—research as flourishing (Cherkowski & Walker, 2017). We were intentionally structuring, or crafting, our research work in ways that opened us up to a mind and heart shift that reflected our belief that what we pay attention to will grow, and that we aimed to pay attention to teacher wellbeing in their work. We were also establishing intentional desires to grow and flourish ourselves, and with our research team.

We saw our research as a set of opportunities to connect authentically and intentionally with our participants as mutual learners and contributors in what we have started to think of as the *pipeline of wellbeing* in schools (Cherkowski & Walker, 2017). This metaphorical pipeline runs through the educational system from early learning settings through the university system, and offers a steady flow of knowledge, practices, resources, and relationships for growing wellbeing for all. Through our research, teaching, and service at the university level, we aim to offer as much as we can to the pipeline, and we appreciatively accept offerings from others as opportunities to grow wellbeing, our own and others', in our educational places and spaces (Cherkowski & Walker, 2017).

We identified four methodological principles of our research on flourishing in schools that provided the foundation for our research process, serving as guiding values and practices for our inquiry flourishing in schools. As you will notice, these pillars of our research into flourishing are reflected in the mindful alignment arts and practices:

- Authentic partnerships—People are at the center of our purpose.
- Appreciative lenses—We see flourishing as potential in all schools.
- Generative dissemination—We hope to share our learning in ways that reflect, inform, and inspire flourishing in all schools.
- Integrative research agenda—We strive to research, teach, and live from a strengths-based, appreciative, positive perspective.

These principles guided us to craft our research processes in schools that built a sense of relationships with our participants, that encouraged each school site to design research processes that reflected their unique school culture and their own interests for understanding what it means to flourish at work. We worked with each school to develop research activities that were research-based, using findings from the literature in the theoretical framework, and that reflected their particular personality, interests, and needs as a teacher culture. For example, one middle school (grades 7–9) worked with us to create a month-long inquiry into flourishing where teachers, who were already grouped into home groups by subjects, would notice and report by email to their group leader any and all moments in their work where they felt well, encouraged, engaged, connected, and inspired in their work. These emails were also sent to us, so that we could track their responses as data for our research. This teaching group enjoyed friendly competition, and so decided to make it a fun game to see which group could collect the most moments of flourishing throughout the month. They described to us that through this research process they felt even more connected to their colleagues in their home groups through sharing all of these important moments in their days, weeks, and months, and that they felt a little happier at work when they took the time to notice, record, and send their moment of flourishing to others in their group. They shared that, through taking the time to notice their own sense of wellbeing, they were starting to pay more attention to the ways they structured the classroom for their students' wellbeing, too. Others shared that they were connecting with their students in a different way now that they were looking for all the moments of goodness in their work.

At the end of the month we celebrated their participation in this research activity and formally announced the winner of the competition at an ice cream sundae reception in the staff room. This culminating meeting reflected the connections that had been built between the teachers, and between us and the teachers, over the course of this activity. We provided them with a written compilation of all their expressions of flourishing as an artifact that they could continue to reflect on and use for their own positive growth and development. One team shared with us that day that they did not even care that they did not win because this inquiry gave them an opportunity to develop stronger connections and appreciation for each other that they might not otherwise have grown (Cherkowski & Walker, under review). While we certainly appreciated the opportunity to collect all the rich narrative data through the month-long email campaign, what resonated even more deeply for us is that this research activity reflected our belief that that we can make a difference through the scholarship and research that we do. We designed a research methodology that empowered us to craft our work of researching flourishing in schools so that we, too, might grow toward a greater sense of flourishing as educational researchers.

As we engaged with educators to understand what it means for them to experience their work from a sense of flourishing, this opened new spaces for conversations about teaching and leading in schools that dug into what matters most to each of us as humans—deep connections, living from passion and purpose, meaningful contributions, and collaborations. When we started paying attention to what makes educators come alive and feel more engaged and enthusiastic in their work, we started to notice all the ways that we also aim to live well with others in our work and in our lives. We have come to understand these varied ways of living well with others at work in schools as flourishing.

Mindful alignment is an ongoing inquiry practice of paying deep attention to self in relation to others and to the world, supported by several arts. Our hope is that, through the literature that we provide to support your learning about mindful alignment, you will find your path toward your flourishing in your own work and life. From this research, we see that educators value opportunities to think about and talk about what helps them to flourish at work and we have also noted that engaging in these positive reflections has provided energy and life during the conversations in ways that then carry over into the rest of their work. Through our work with educators, we are learning that an intentional and deliberate focus on what contributes to thriving requires support and encouragement. However, this is not always the default mode for teachers' reflections. Although there is strong benefit and payoffs for attending to the positive, we know that there is a competing and often stronger need to pay attention to the negative—what Kim Cameron (2008) calls the "negativity bias." As a founding scholar in positive organizational studies, he highlights that we should work to override a natural tendency to pay attention to the negative in our environment. He finds that we can override this negativity bias and attend more intentionally to the positive in ways that create what he calls "a virtuous cycle" or "positive deviance"— acts that go above and beyond in the direction of positive. In our research we are actively paying attention to stories of positive deviance in the work of teaching and learning.

In the next chapter, we explore the first aspect of mindful alignment: paying attention to wellbeing. We describe some of the ways we can open up new avenues for the personal and professional development of wellbeing for ourselves and others. We consider several theories and practices for attunement of wellbeing, and then focus on the art of attuning to disciplines of engagement and abstinence as a practice for becoming mindfully aware of the experiences that make up our lives, and assessing the alignment of these with our sense of purpose and our goals for ourselves. We describe the value of paying attention to wellbeing as our sense of wholeness and learning to grow our awareness of how we can craft mindful alignment.

Chapter Two

Wellbeing as Wholeness

The first aspect of mindful alignment is a prioritized attention on wellbeing as a holistic expression of our humanness. This holistic view of body, mind, and spirit is essential to our thinking about true alignment. Of course there are many ways to understand the distinct and yet connected components that make up the human being. For some, there is the material part (body/flesh) and the spiritual part (soul/spirit). Some others hold to the view that we are body, soul, and spirit. Still others view humans as having body and soul facets that are a united whole. There is also the Cartesian dualism that helps us to make sense of the separation of mind and body (or the difference between our mind and our brain). These distinctions and their nuances may be important for some purposes, but for our design these point to extending our vocabulary and embracing a more complex humanity. We think that having vocabulary and experiences that pay attention to each and all aspects of our being has critical implications for our wellbeing. Obviously, reminding ourselves of the various facets of our makeup isn't sufficient without a plan or schema of various tools, technologies, or approaches that can be taken to establish and sustain our wellbeing. As we will describe later in the chapter, we call these habits "disciplines," and offer a practice of mindful awareness to the disciplines of engagement and abstinence as a practice, or art, for mindful alignment.

THE PRIORITY OF FOCUSING ON ONE'S OWN WELLBEING

We sometimes forget the vital role that wellbeing plays in terms of our capacities to sustain our service to others. This may sound simple or even simplistic, but in our personal and research experiences, the incidence of forgetfulness seems higher than it ought to be. As we consider a mindful approach to a professional's development, we need to encourage and support one another to look after our own wellbeing in addition to our caring for others. Wellbeing has been described by some as related to psychological health, personal, domestic, and work satisfaction, and the capacity to function well and live in harmony and congruence. When life isn't experienced as congruent, then educators can become inauthentic and wear masks that cover their sense of messiness, ineptness, and disorder. Such duplicitous living does not equate with living as an educator who expresses excellence of character and high virtue. To live an aligned and authentic life, professionals need to match their passions and their behaviors with their clear values; their habits with their reliability, predictability, and consistency; their compassion with their heartfelt convictions; and their social situations with their high view of connections and concentric circles of relationships (both distant and close).

We are reminded of the aircraft stewards' safety instructions before take-off, to put on one's own oxygen mask first and then to look after others. Self-care is vital. For an educator to provide continuing and sustained service, she must be healthy in each dimension of her life. There are many ways and measures for personal wellness. Basically, wellness is often explained in terms of self-care: healthy exercise and nutrition, adequate sleep, meaningful work, and positive relationships. To be well is to have found our balance and mastery over the habits of life that sustain our physical, mental-emotional, social, and spiritual wellbeing. To do so enables us to "live to the full," a good life. As a former counselor, one of our writing team members recollects the advice of a more senior mentor who suggested that more than half of the counseling clients were predictably helped by asking them questions about the most basic of their life patterns: Are you exercising, eating well, sleeping well, and relating well? Once they had gauged the physical, mental, emotional-social, and spiritual barometers or thermostats, then the most practical counseling would entail encouraging or exhorting them to make efforts and to find resources to help them to sleep well, eat well, exercise regularly, and to generally be kind to themselves and others. Without being too sanguine here (we know that life circumstances can be profoundly difficult), we might ask: Could it be that some of our profound issues are rooted in our failure to align to some of the most basic of life-sustaining practices (sleeping, eating, exercising, and being kind)?

For educators, it is both possible and all too common to neglect certain aspects of one's wellbeing with the excuse that there are more pressing issues. This behavior is to the ultimate detriment of both health and performance. In our experience this is the MO (modus operandi or method of operation) for many educators. As we describe above, it is crucial to appreciate that we are multidimensional beings and that we must give attention to our maintenance and fitness in each and all of the dimensions of our lives. As a person becomes physically unfit or unwell, undue fatigue and physical stress begin to affect their capacities and their endurance, and other dimensions of wellbeing may also collapse. Educators will know about this in their own experiences and in the lives of those they've worked with. Routine health check-ups, balance of diet, exercise, adequate sleep, compliance with medical advice, abstaining from unhealthy practices, and living a well-paced life will all contribute to physical wellness.

Like us, you have certainly heard the well-known mantras that physical wellbeing is about making daily smart choices in the areas of diet, exercise, and sleep. Rath and Harter (2010) assert that, "Physical wellbeing is about having good health and enough energy to get things done on a daily basis" (p. 155). As a former health educator, one of our writing team members remembers adding to this definition of fitness that it isn't just about having enough energy to get done what one needs to do by the end of the day, *but also* to have sufficient reserve to handle periodic unplanned or emergent calls upon our physical capacities. People with high physical wellbeing feel better, learn and think more effectively, have more energy, live longer, have an active lifestyle, and can handle the unexpected physical demands of life—from time to time. Diet has a direct correlation to energy, longevity, cognition, and mental health. Though genetics influences our physical health, wise health choices contribute to controlling the expression of your genetic makeup. Rath and Harter (2010) write, "So even if you have a gene that predisposes you to a chronic disease, there are things you can do to either silence or amplify the expression of that gene" (p. 73). Though sometimes we are more educated than obedient to what we know, we all know that exercise contributes to elevated levels of physical and mental health. Energy levels rise, stress decreases, and moods elevate in educators who exercise for at least twenty minutes a day. Indeed, exercise can be effective for eliminating fatigue. Quality sleep is a major contributor to physical wellbeing because sleep improves our mood, increases energy, and enables us to better concentrate and learn. Rath and Harter (2010) affirm that "Scientists are discovering that we learn and make connections *more effectively when we are asleep* than we do when we are awake. Each night of sleep allows our brain to process what we learned the day before" (p. 82). Also, when people sleep on a decision or a problem, they are more likely to be successful in solving the problem and making the best decision after that good sleep. The amount of sleep people need for optimal benefits to health, memory, appearance, and wellbeing varies from between seven to eight hours. Lack of sleep increases the likelihood of weight gain and even of catching a cold.

Rath and Harter (2010) offer the notion of career wellbeing as an aspect of our lives that helps us to further frame what it is that we should give attention to sustaining. They suggest that this type of wellbeing encompasses our enjoyment of work and the development of deep purposes attached to our vocation (or calling) to serve. A career plan will include our hope to make a difference, fulfill a cause, or attain to significant and particular life goals. Rath and Harter (2010) contend, as do we, that every human being needs to have something meaningful to do and something to look forward to. Often in our research with educators, we have been inspired by the responses to our question: "What gets you up and to school most morning?" In other words, what makes you tick and what motivates or drives you? The stories and the deeply held convictions and aspirations are so energizing to hear. How do you respond to these kinds of questions?

We advocate that educators develop their own career or professional platform. A platform is something you stand on, a way to see further, or a set of self-understandings that help scaffold our day-to-day decisions. This professional platform may be generated by developing a professional mission statement and articulating one's key values. We suggest that verifying your own values, beliefs, convictions, and life principles; articulating your own ethical grid about what is good, bad, proper, improper, right, wrong, virtuous, and vicious; determining to learn everyday about how to better weigh various perspectives on issues; choosing to act with integrity and through diligent action; evaluating your own growth in terms of what is truly important to you as a professional; and developing the capacity to "talk and act out loud" about these values which become both subjective and objective professional responsibilities, will help platform development.

To develop one's platform, some educators have found responding to several questions to be a good starting point:

1. Who are your models in life—images of professional educators or leaders—and their qualities?
2. What is your professional mission and how do your strengths relate to this mission?
3. As a professional educator, what is the difference you wish to make?
4. What are the professional convictions and causes that matter most to you?
5. What are your beliefs about motivating, influencing, relating, serving and leading others?
6. How do you intend to model and mentor those in your circle of personal and professional influence to become all they wish to become?

Those with high career wellbeing have something to look forward to when they wake up every morning, because they know in their heart of hearts that they will be using their strengths to do work that both interests them (aligns with their passions) and makes a positive difference in the lives of others. Those with high professional career wellbeing act and think in ways that are engaging, meaningful, and interesting. Rath and Harter (2010) find that people who enjoy their work also thrive in personal time. They write, "They love their work so much that it is closely aligned with—and can't help but spill over into—their personal lives" (p. 22).

So, we've suggested that being actively engaged in one's work will contribute to general happiness and wellbeing. Those who are not engaged in their work often watch the clock, are less happy, and experience more stress but get happier toward the end of the workday. Put another way, being disengaged in our work settings contributes to the increased possibility of being diagnosed with depression. It is interesting to us that nearly two-thirds of the people who reach their 50s do not want to retire. Rath and Harter (2010) also maintain that "compared to those who do *not* get to focus on what they do best, people who have the opportunity to use their strengths are *six times* as likely to be engaged in their jobs and more than *three times* as likely to report having an excellent quality of life" (p. 28). Having fun at work, using one's strengths, and doing something meaningful leads to career wellbeing—and retiring from such a positive environment is difficult for many people.

Educators who are well have cultivated an understanding of themselves—what motivates, what depletes, what energizes, and what drains them. Emotionally healthy educators know what triggers the best and worst in themselves and experience appropriate emotional responsiveness as life happens around and to them and others. They have the ability to identify, express, and empathize with feelings of anger, frustration, fear, sadness, hope, love, humor, and joy, and can deal with (manage/cope) each of these emotional states and signals in productive ways, especially as life brings challenges to them and others.

We also suggest that the capacity for wellbeing for a professional educator is strongly limited or unleashed by their spiritual wellbeing. Wellbeing is holistic and involves attention to matters of the mind, body, heart, and spirit. For us, the spiritual nature of wellbeing is about connecting our ever-maturing sense of our personhood, our identity, and our core values with profound questions about our lives and what it means to be a human being. Our spiritedness thrives when there is room in our lives to connect these "deeper" life questions, which might include matters of love, suffering, death, mystery, the natural world, to our day-to-day explorations. Parker Palmer (1999a) offers an example of teachers who teach in ways that honor the spirited nature of learning, writing, "I know a geography teacher who asks students to keep a journal of their daily interactions with rocks, an assignment that initially strikes them as odd but eventually helps them understand how intertwined their lives are with the earth" (p. 4). We believe that human spirit is always present, and so it is not something we need to bring into our lives, but rather something we need to honor and respect within ourselves and each other by carving out space to converse and explore in these ways.

We believe that when we share the spiritual connections we make to the world with each other a deep sense of community can emerge.

Educator colleagues will vary greatly in terms of how articulate and thoughtful they are about this dimension of wellbeing, how dogmatic they are in terms of their understandings, or how explicit and conscious they are with respect to the language, practices, and expression of spirituality. This dimension of wellbeing is likely to call for more conscious mutual respect and room for wider expressions of understandings than other aspects of well-being. Of course there are varieties of philosophic and religious definitions, descriptions, and stipulations that mediate our understandings and apprecia-tions of spiritual wellbeing. For our purposes, we would offer that, at the very least, spiritual wellness is about our inner life and its relationship with our own capacities and our relationships with the wider world.

WHAT ABOUT HAPPINESS?

"Happiness," as we are using the term, is the state produced by weaving our engagement in activities that matter and that are fulfilling, fruitful, and con-sistent with our deeply held values, interests, and beliefs. This is the state of wellbeing that experiences fulfillment in both the journey, as well as in the anticipation of the joy that comes from achieving various stations and mile-stones along the way. The joy of achieving the legacy-leaving and signature contributions (large or small) for which we, as educators, were designed to make is what it means to be happy with one's lot in life. To know who I am, as a person with gender, culture, ethnic, state, clan, vocational fit, and famil-ial identity is to be at peace with myself and with the world. To be comfort-able in one's own skin; this is what it means to be happy, to have a sense of being self-determed, and to excercise governance over all that ought to be rightfully in one's control. This is a good thing. Autonomy (freedom), com-petency (to attain goals), and efficacy (a sense that one's doing can make a difference), are normal experiences and point to the good life. These are the elements of what has been called self-determination theory (Deci & Ryan, 1999).

Humans are complicated and dynamic beings. There are both universal and unique aspects of our design. Each educator is best advised to become familiar with the general dimensions and spheres of wellbeing and then to constantly challenge themselves to attain to the status and realizations of subjective and objective wellbeing. In ancient times, the Greek philosophers wrestled with these ideas about how to live a good life. The revered teachers of that time, such as Socrates and Plato, were known to have an understand-ing of their truest selves, and their capacity to live from this place of authen-ticity was seen as the wisdom required to serve as a teacher. Indeed, Aristotle gave us the Greek word for flourishing—*eudemonia*—pointing to that important journey of self-discovery that we all ought to follow in our lives, as we seek to discover and live into the truest or most divine within for the purpose of contributing to improvement of the common and highest good. The goal was not to seek pleasure for immediate gratification, or what was known as hedonism. Rather, living a good life was to be in the service of contributing to others' abilities to also live a good life and to contribute to the common and higher good. Aristotle maintained that human beings have the *desire* to be happy.

Jean Vanier (2001), the founder of the L'Arche communities, asserts that the great aspiration of men and women is to know happiness or the fullness of life. He says that to be truly human means "becoming as perfectly accomplished as possible. . . . Accomplishment derives from the exercise of the most perfect activity: that of seeking the truth in all things, shunning lies and illusion, acting in accordance with justice, transcending oneself to act for the good of others in society" (pp. xiv–xv), and that "we human beings are drawn to ends; we desire them, we want to possess them, consume them, be one with them; we want to look at them, contemplate them, take our delight in them" (p. 6). Vanier (2001) illustrats this by saying that "Just as a seed planted in the earth will grow to fullness of life, provided it is watered, so a human being aspires to his own fullness of life" (p. 196). As the plant needs water, the human needs knowledge, choices, and even struggles. As we develop as persons and professionals, we strive to thrive and to attain increasingly more qualitative happiness. We experience conflicts, tensions, and these engage our desire for more refined and improved attainments of happiness and experiences of flourishing.

Spitzer (2000) provides a helpful description of this in his depiction of four levels of happiness. The first level of happiness operates at the physical or material level (akin to hedonism) where possession, sensual gratification, relieving physical thirst, hunger, pain, and physical urgings are handled just as quickly as possible. In the longstanding formulation of this type of immediate gratification, the person's objective is to maximize pleasure and minimize pain. It is primarily focused on an obligation to look after oneself. As the law of diminishing returns works itself out, a person experiences the need to continue to step up the efforts and means to get pleasure and to avoid pain, emptiness, boredom, fear of loss, and loneliness. Spitzer indicates that the vicious cycle of dissatisfaction with the inadequacy of Happiness 1, pushes us to pursue Happiness 2, where we want to gain the advantage over others, to promote ourselves, to have power and control, and to achieve or attain, and, in doing so, focus on short-term ego gratification. It is helpful to look at these levels as developmental. Of course, the stability that comes with goal attainment, successes, recognition of our work, and efforts to gain a comparative advantage over others through possessions, popularity, and power is understandable and pursuit-worthy. Just as our healthy development out of "stuck-ness" at the Happiness 1 level is spurred on by a crisis of dissatisfaction, so, too, do we come to a place of yearning for more in terms of our happiness. Happiness 3, according to Spitzer, sets us on the journey of replacing the "comparison game" with efforts to look for the good beyond ourselves, to make the world around us a better place. We have this innate desire to have a cause, to enhance humanity, to make a significant difference, to embody the ideals of justice, temperance, truth, beauty, wisdom, courage, and love. And we find ourselves working on behalf of others with a long-term and sustainable view of making a positive difference (i.e., leaving a legacy). All three of these levels have their joys, accumulative and complementary benefits, and put "wind in our sails." There comes a time when our pursuit of meaning and happiness begins to uncover the natural desire of humans for self-transcendence and full self-actualization ("yes"—think Abraham Maslow and *Third Force Psychology*, or Victor Frankl and *Man's Search for Meaning*). In Happiness 4, there is a pursuit of the greatest common good—the higher good, exchanging ultimate meaning, and being entirely "at home" with oneself, others, and a higher spiritual force. The ethic of desire (Aristotle) uses discernment in order to distinguish between the superficial and the more profound (between H1/H2 and H3/H4) and to "identify and shed light on what is in our inner depths" (Vanier, 2012, 7). As he understands Aristotle, Vanier suggests that humans seek the supreme good that is happiness (H4). As individual educators deliberately identify happiness, seek it, make good choices, and understand that it may take a lifetime to achieve, they progress in their state of happiness. Happiness can describe our current and future (aspired for) states.

The self-prescriptions for achieving wellbeing and the state of happiness will be uniquely determined by many personal, situational, and pre-conditioned factors. We know that an educator must be able to lead themselves, to take charge of their own wellbeing, and to do all they can to lead those in their care into the same state of soundness of body, mind, emotions, relations, and spirit. Professional educators need to choose to be healthy—to take whatever steps are needed to regularly assess their own fitness in order to be able to lead others to wellbeing. Put another way, the challenge is to be happy and well ourselves, such as we are able to offer a safe example for others to follow. The new generation of educators are challenged with helping students to succeed as authentically healthy and happy. This is a complex challenge, requiring educators to attend to various dimensions of wellbeing at one time. Single dimensional educators who are unhealthy in other dimensions will not be able to sustain their leadship of others. They will also be vulnerable to compromise, unnecessary fragility, and even corruption. Happy educators produce healthy and happy environments for their constituents. We sometimes think of an educator's efforts to seek their own wellbeing as "soul keeping." The whole person certainly is a complex being—wonderfully made and beyond our complete understanding. In the next section, we describe a practice, an art, for attending to the multidimensionality of wellbeing through attuning to disciplines of engagement and abstinence. These are ways of noticing and nurturing opportunities for growing wellbeing across the many dimensions of work and life.

MINDFUL ART PRACTICE FOR WELLBEING: PAYING ATTENTION TO DISCIPLINES

As this chapter was being written, the season for New Year's resolutions had sufficiently passed by such that most of the intentions for new starts, crucial lifestyle changes, and life-altering "should-do"s had faded into the second month of the year and the distractions of "life back to the usual." Depending on who you listen to, the general efficacy of New Year's resolutions is quite limited. Our congratulations to those who consistently beat the odds and who have experienced transformation by choosing to make a change; the desired change and the source of the change has been sustained. We celebrate this with you. It is likely that you had one thing (something doable that you wanted badly) to do or change. "Less is more" when it comes to resolutions. It is likely that those we are celebrating with did not have three or four such resolutions. The chances of making more than one significant change at a time is slight, at best. One thing that we know about human will-power is that it is both weak and strong. Making one thing the main thing, and concentrating on that one thing, can work for us if we plan to succeed. So make a wellbeing resolution. Resolve and determine to disturb your status quo and habituate a new practice that adds value to you and others.

Develop an Inventory of Disciplines for Educator Wellbeing

Personalizing practices to suit your own goals, intentions, and life contexts is a sustainable approach to developing your wellbeing. For this practice we have designed a template for you to explore your own understanding and ideas about ways to attend to your wellbeing. This is a brief inventory of disciplines for educator wellbeing.

A discipline, whether focused on the physical, emotional, intellectual, or spiritual aspects of our wellbeing, is meant to enable us to do what we are able to do and find life balance. Discipline is about self-care and self-mastery; it has to do with exercising control over what we can control and letting go of what we can't control. Educators who know and follow the discipline themselves are more likely to serve as leaders for others to grow their own wellbeing. To displace unhealthy habits, compulsions or obsessions, we exercise certain habits/disciplines designed to establish and sustain our health-fulness and our happiness. Again, there is a discipline to the notion of "less is more." Various traditions from ancient to modern, religious and not relig-ious, have tried and tested methods and approaches to disciplines of spirit, mind and body. In the section that follows we are going to present a number of disciplines, or practices, that may resonate with the reader. Again, we do not intend to be comprehensive or prescriptive at all, but simply to name a few categories of practice that have been found to be helpful to others. Of course there are many, many ways to experience these disciplines. We sim-ply want to put these out there because it is our view that mindful practice is an expansive canvas for us to write on.

One way of seeing disciplines is to consider some as disciplines of en-gagement and others as disciplines of abstinence. These are inner disciplines to be cultivated by deliberate practice and choice-making. As indicated, a discipline is an activity within our power that enables us to accomplish what we cannot do by direct or casual effort. We know that we can't be at all sure about our future lives and circumstances. As researchers and educators, we have found that much of what we experience in our lives is *not* within the realm of our control or governance. We desire other people to do certain things and they will either do what we expect or they will disappoint us. We listen to the news, and so much that is commendable, as well as what is despicable is far away, removed from our immediate realm and beyond our reach. A discipline, at least the way we are framing the concept, is about our taking charge of that which we can exercise control over by our choices. For example, our breathing is automatic in the sense that the respiratory center in my brain stem continuously, involuntarily directs the function. I can exercise some conscious control over my breathing, with focus and certain interven-tions. This slight foothold or intermediary stepping into the body and mind space, and the awareness of my breathing, is something I can do, with prac-tice. Breathing awareness and associated techniques are fundamental to mindfulness practices. Our point is that breathing is a function within the realm of our partial governance, and discipline is a pattern of behavior where we choose to do or not do what we have rulership over. Our bodies, minds, emotions, and volition are within the scope of our control or self-control. We can exercise willpower to override habits or behaviors or feelings or thoughts or choices; not necessarily easily, but with practice. We can change behav-iors, feelings, thoughts, and choice-making patterns. This is an inside-out phenomenon. We won't address brain plasticity here, but suffice it to say that the human brain can reorganize itself in some rather incredible and life-altering ways.

Sometimes discipline is about suppressing some basic desires, restraining natural inclinations, or not just "going with the flow." Other times it is about risking the unfamiliar, changing one's orientation, attitude, or first judgments. It is about doing the right, good, virtuous, beneficial, and proper thing when it might be easier to do otherwise. The kind of disciplines we are thinking about here for educators have to do with being the kind of person we want to be when we are at our best so that our potential is fully realized, and an example that is safe for others to follow. It is not about stoic obedience to a set of rules, but rather we have disciplines in mind that require discernment, an openness to personal transformation, and some measured appetite for doing things slightly differently, being patient with ourselves, and enduring a bit of discomfort. Those who know how to sail well are able to sense the wind and its encounter with the boat and the water; they discern through practice to adjust the disposition of the sails accordingly. They engage and they disengage with the wind depending on the preferred destination. So it is with the disciplines that we present here.

For this art of mindful alignment we are providing a selective list of disciplines and encourage you to reflect on these in your own words. Feel free to add other disciplines as you consider your own circumstances and dispositions, and as you seek to cultivate these. We also encourage you to take some time reflecting on how these disciplines might show up in your life. As you engage in this practice, what you attend to will grow more and as you grow your awareness, you will begin to a notice greater degree of alignment in your wellbeing. Our descriptions are not meant to be limiting or definitive but, rather, to provide a window into some of your own disciplines. Our descriptions are illustrative and roughly articulated to allow you to consider your own descriptions, interpretations, and adaptations.

Educators thrive on personally meaningful or significant practices that enhance and sustain their wellbeing, transform their experiences of work and ultimately benefit the wellbeing and happiness of others. The mindful art of attending to disciplines and the practical development of wellbeing priorities only scratch the surface of the well-worn practices from ancient through contemporary times. We are hoping that the educators who read this book are willing to stretch into some new and useful disciplines of wellbeing and healthfulness. An awareness of some options beyond our current practices may be helpful, and we encourage readers to seek out a variety of practices and routines that resonate with them as supports for growing and maintaining wellbeing.

While we may have focused on individual wellbeing in this chapter, we know from research and from our own lived experiences that we are social beings who need connection, attachment, and a sense of belonging with others to thrive. In the next chapter, we grow our understanding of a holistic sense of wellbeing to highlight the importance of positive relationships as the second aspect of attention for growing and sustaining mindful alignment.

Table 2.1.   Descriptions of Selected Disciplines for Mindful Alignment

Descriptions of Selected Disciplines	*What My Practice of this Discipline Might Look Like*
Solitude is about getting away or "escaping" or retreating. It can be for a weekend, a few minutes or hours. It can be experienced by finding a place to "be alone" or getting away from everybody or is some way that works—finding peaceful quiet. This discipline is more difficult than we sometimes think.	**Example:** Each weekend I look for small, even just a few minutes opportunities to find time alone. I might take longer way to the mailbox or when I am doing a chore I focus on and enjoy the quiet. I get some time apart from others; some time for myself. I shut down my cell phone and settle into some disconnecting with others but strongly connect with myself and my thoughts.
Listening is about clearing our minds from distractions that might keep us from being wide-awake to the voices of others or ourselves. Being fully present and actively attending to another person such that we make space for what they have to say and we concentrate on the meaning of their words.	
Celebrating is about seeking opportunities to honor ourselves and others. It nurtures the fine art of joyful occasions and recognitions. Celebrations commemorate and enjoy what has worked and this discipline makes a place for gratitude and joy, such as displaces negativity and cynicism.	
Journaling is about keeping a simple record of our experiences, feelings, thoughts, and reflections. The practice puts words to our lives and enhances the focus, clarity, expression, and organization of what is meaningful, difficult, and delightful to us.	
Praying is about having a conversation with an unseen Other in a way that expresses our thanksgiving, makes known our needs and asks for help or enjoys the companionship of the Other.	
Service is about choosing to give our time, talents, energy, or resources for the benefit of others. Sacrificing or exchanging what we have or could have in order that others might have. Service is about cheerfully giving to others.	

Descriptions of Selected Disciplines	What My Practice of this Discipline Might Look Like

Slowing is about parenthesizing the demands of life by deliberately changing our speed and pace (getting into a different lane). It is about making space for recalibrating one's sense of urgency and re-evaluating what is important. It is about drinking more deeply from the wells that replenish and refresh us. As we slow down, we courageously say "no" more often and without guilt, so we can say "yes" to what is more generative and life-giving.

Forgiving is about letting go and choosing not to be held captive to hurt and injury inflicted by the words, deeds, or omissons of others. It is about releasing self and health consuming bitterness, grudge, anger and the weight of obligation to see justice done. It is the decision to not be defined by our wounds and the offenses of another. It is about finding grace and peace to move on and through an undeserved difficulty.

Stillness is about doing nothing on purpose. It is about sitting with ourself and quieting our body and our mind in order to recreate and simply "be." It is about making time to re-set our reactive impulses to connect with one's true self and to create margins or white spaces for relaxation.

Simplicity is about acknowledging that anxiety and fear are tied to our acquiring and our unfettered appetites and attachments. Simplicity is about asking what is the minimum we need rather than succumbing to the pressure to get as much as we can. Simplicity is about focusing on what is most important and letting go of accumulated "stuff."

Descriptions of Selected Disciplines	***What My Practice of this Discipline Might Look Like***

Fasting is about going without, delaying gratification, or breaking away from attachments that may be mastering us (rather than the other way around). It is about reversing the control of things over our lives (obsessions, addictions, co-dependencies) and resolving to be self-controlled and temperate, even when faced with the strongest of temptations and triggers. It is about deferring to gain back freedom and autonomy.

Silence is about being quiet, patient, waiting, and temporarily abstaining from speaking to allow for inner dialogue or internal focus. It is about choosing not to fill the air with our outer voice in order to pay attention to our inner stirrings.

Confessing is about admitting to oneself or to an Other that we have missed the mark, blown it, that we have disappointed expectations or obligations through what we have done or left undone. It is about witnessing and agreeing that we are decidedly imperfect. It is about coming clean and agreeing with internal (conscience) or external standards that we were wrong. We say that we are sorry, that we are choosing to do better next time and that we seek forgiveness for our offenses.

Mourning is about feeling deep empathy and concern for the loss suffered or pain experienced by others. It gives us permission to grieve our own losses. It is giving ourselves permission to be touched by the hurt experienced by others or to be vulnerable to our won sorrows.

Laughing is about seeing the bright side, enjoying the company of others, not taking ourselves so seriously and deciding to enjoy life and humor. It is about relishing the absurd, taking a break from judging and stress. It is about being out loud with our joy.

Descriptions of Selected Disciplines	What My Practice of this Discipline Might Look Like
Encouraging is about realizing that because words have the power to destroy or give life that we will find ways to embolden others with kindness and look for the good in people and circumstances.	
Ending is about figuring out what aspects of our lives are no longer adding value to us and others; then moving on. It is about finishing, abandoning, or stopping that which is stale or dated but still drawing energy or attention from us. It is about letting go of the older to make room for the new.	

Chapter Three

Positive Relationships

This chapter is about our mindful awareness of the complex nature of the relationships in our lives. As we adjust the scope of our awareness of relationships, we want to assert that the act of listening transforms. We suggest that listening is a gateway; it is the connection between the subjective and the collective, and it is a way to cultivate deep and fulfilling access to the benefits of relationality. Mindful awareness of relationships can be seen as an act of love or compassion. We need to listen to ourselves and be kind to ourselves, just as we need to listen to others and exercise compassion with them. Love, or positivity resonance (Fredrickson, 2013), has benefits for self and others as "micro-moments of love carry irrepressible ripple effects across whole social networks, helping each person who experiences positivity resonance to grow and in turn touch and uplift the lives of countless others" (p. 37). Though all positive emotions provide benefits—broadens one's mindset (becoming more flexible, attuned to others, creative, wise) and build resourcefulness (more knowledgeable, more resilient, more socially integrated, healthier)—love is the supreme emotion that makes us come most fully alive. Fredrickson (2013) assertes that love goes beyond contributing to a positive feeling. In fact, love can be a life-giving source of energy, sustenance, and health. Love, from the physical perspective of the body, can alter our biochemicals. As Fredrickson claims, "the love you do or do not experience today may quite literally change key aspects of your cellular architecture next season and next year—cells that affect your physical health, your vitality, and your overall wellbeing" (2013, p. 4). In this chapter, we outline several key aspects of positive relationships and then provide a description and practice of the mindful art of listening for attuning to mindful alignment of positive relationships.

POSITIVE EMOTIONS

Feeling a sense of wellbeing includes positive emotions, or feelings, described by Seligman (2011) and Fredrickson (2004) as pleasure, warmth, comfort, joy, interest, contentment, and love. There are tremendous benefits associated with experiencing positive emotions including the broadening of the educator's capacity to learn, be optimistic, flexible, and creative in their thinking. Experiencing emotional and physical resilience and love can undo the effects of stress. In other words, as Kesebir and Diener (2008) state, "positive affect and general wellbeing produce a state from which individuals can confidently explore the environment and approach new goals, thus allowing them to build important personal resources" (p. 63). Positive emotions affect brain function and behaviors that benefit aspects of living successfully. Achor (2011) writes, "they [positive emotions] help us build more intellectual, social, and physical resources we can rely on in the future" (p. 44). The chemicals dopamine and serotonin, released through positive emotions, enhance the learning centers of the brain, enabling the organization of information, memory, thinking speed, and creative and analytical thought. When people are in a good mood, "they get primed for creativity and innovation" (Achor, 2011, p. 45). Positive feelings heighten and broaden one's thought-action repertoires and build intellectual, psychological, social, and physical resources over time.

Positive emotions influence learning, just as learning contributes to one's sense of wellbeing. In other words, as we experience positive emotions in our professional learning, we are more able to learn and grow. We activate our capacities to broaden and build our learning in that moment and we will feel a sense of wellbeing in our achievement of learning. This contributes to a virtuous cycle of learning and wellbeing. Some of the beneficial thought processes associated with experiencing positive emotion include being flexible, attentive, creative, integrative, open to information, and efficient. Fredrickson also noted that those with positive affect have the ability to integrate diverse material and they also register an increase in brain dopamine levels (2004, p. 1370).

Fredrickson's (2004) *broaden-and-build* theory of positive emotions may be described as the ability of positive emotions to "*broaden* peoples' momentary thought-action repertoires and *build* their enduring personal resources" (p. 1369). As an educator experiences the positive emotions of joy, interest, contentment, and love, for example, Fredrickson determines that there is a *broadening* within one's momentary thought-action repertoire. Fredrickson (2004) explains that "joy sparks the urge to play, interest sparks the urge to explore, contentment sparks the urge to savour and integrate, and love sparks a recurring cycle of each of these urges within safe, close relationships" (p. 1367). Thus, through these positive emotions, the person's physical, intellectual, social, and psychological resources are *built* up as novel and creative actions are experienced and discovered and where ideas and social bonds are enhanced. Fredrickson asserts, "These various thought-action tendencies—to play, to explore, or to savour and integrate—each represents ways that positive emotions broaden habitual modes of thinking or acting" (p. 1369). In turn, these resources are "banked," or reserved, and can later be drawn upon to increase coping or survival success.

Not only do positive emotions produce wellbeing and optimal functioning during the present moments of a person's life, but Fredrickson (2004) argues that, over the long-term, positive emotions are "a means to achieving psychological growth and improved psychological and physical wellbeing" (p. 1367). As educators experience positive emotions, they are able to transform or change themselves, "becoming more creative, knowledgeable, resilient, socially integrated and healthy individuals" (Fredrickson, 2004, p. 1369). Positive emotions are powerful sparks that ignite wellbeing and flourishing in life.

Fredrickson's research of the broaden-and-build theory found "that distinct positive emotions widen the array of thoughts and actions that come to mind" (2004, p. 1370). In contrast, negative emotions narrow peoples' attention and thought-action repertoire, resulting in less learning. Positive emotions are linked to more pro-social behavior and less hyperactive and/or aggressive behavior. As such, it would be beneficial for students and staff to pay attention to their thoughts, their feelings, and their sensations as they learn and play, and to choose actions and behaviors that fit with pro-social and personal interests. Ben-Shahar (2008) extolls the benefits of being a curious, inquisitive person for this leads to more learning resulting in greater happiness, more creativity, positive relationships, and higher levels of success.

Achor (2011) states, "What we spend our time and mental energy focusing on can indeed become our reality" (p. 12). Experiencing positive relationships and positive learning experiences with others creates a sense of wellbeing in ourselves and others, and the act of contributing to increasing someone else's sense of happiness increases our own even more. Finding ways to cultivate positive relationships and to experience positive moments together is really the wellbeing gift that keeps on giving; the benefits continue to multiply. As we have described, the practice of improving our wellbeing is not only about our feelings, our thoughts, and our moods; it is also a more physiological experience, one that is physically experienced in our bodies. For example, Ben-Shahar (2009) reminds us that "a smile will bring about a more positive feeling, whereas a frown will make us feel worse. In fact, we can improve our mood at almost any point by simply smiling, or better, laughing" (p. 116). We live in and through a physical body, and our body can provide an invaluable source of learning about wellbeing, our own and others, as we pay attention. As we will describe in this chapter, there are benefits to wellbeing that improve our physical selves, our bodies, and paying attention to the body is another opportunity to gain a mindful awareness of how we are sensing or physically experiencing an alignment of our values with our behaviors.

Happy people are friendly and extend trust, leading to more opportunities for engaging in social experiences given that "positive mood also enhances interest in social and prosocial activities, increases liking for other people, and leads to more intimate self-disclosures in social interactions" (Tov & Diener, 2008, p. 161). This idea that the benefits of positive emotions and relationships was linked in Marks's (2011) study where he observed that giving to others increased happiness and contributed to a sense of meaning in one's life. The participants were significantly happier spending one hundred dollars on others compared to those who spent the money on themselves. Being both generous and altruistic, in attitude and behavior, resulted in positive benefits, not only for one's own wellbeing but also for the beneficiaries. Indeed, being charitable and grateful are distinct ways to increase one's wellbeing. Love, experienced in and through relationships with others, influences how one feels, thinks, acts, and becomes with self and others. It creates virtuous cycles leading to more health, happiness, and wisdom (Fredrickson, 2004; Haidt, 2006).

DEVELOPING POSITIVE RELATIONSHIPS WITH OTHERS

In his positive psychological research on flourishing, Seligman (2011) found that friends and social relationships are valuable and important to one's happiness. Indeed, this is consistent with ancient wisdom, expressed by Aristotle as a belief that "no one would choose to live without friends, even if he had all the other goods" (Kesebir & Diener, 2008, p. 69) and Epicurus who maintained that "of all the things that wisdom provides to help one live one's entire life in happiness, the greatest by far is the possession of friendship" (p. 69). Contemporary researchers corroborate these views. In all instances, happy people have vibrant social relationships where quality and quantity of friendships are evidenced. As one study suggests, "good social relationships may be the single most important source of happiness" (Kesibir & Diener, 2008, p. 69).

Houston (1996) argues that happiness is not a product nor a personal achievement. Rather, "happiness is the fruit of a gifted life, of goodness received from others, and love given and shared. Happiness can only come our way when we have a strong life in relationship with others" (p. 8). Houston, too, maintains that happiness has a strong social component. As foreshadowed in chapter 2, and in particular from the work of Jean Vanier, one of the critical aspects of happiness is that "happiness can only be complete when it is given to others. . . . It can never be grasped selfishly for our own sake, but must be shared. We simply cannot hold on to happiness. We have to give it away before we, and others, can truly enjoy it" (Houston, 1996, p. 14). Numerous studies strongly assert that positive and supportive social relationships and a sense of belonging are fundamental to wellbeing. Diener and Seligman (2004) affirm that "people need social bonds in committed relationships, not simply interactions with strangers, to experience wellbeing" (p. 237).

Researchers have also shown that trusting relationships are critical for the development of happiness. Layard (2005) asserts that "living where you can trust others makes a clear difference to your happiness" (p. 69). Where students and staff members engage as a community and are accountable to one another in an atmosphere of trust, a sense of belonging is heightened, which inspires engagement and investment in the school's purposes and endeavors. Fostering the feeling of belonging is important because the need to belong is a basic and pervasive human drive. Belonging and acceptance are linked to increased school participation, a positive orientation towards school and teachers, pro-social behavior, and higher expectations for one's own success and behavior. In our flourishing school case studies, students' and educators' feelings of belonging were evidenced as they participated in small group work, understood that their voices were heard, and indicated that they knew that they were cared for at work.

As the experience of trust contributes to a sense of wellbeing, so too do positive emotions contribute to a sense of trust. Tov and Diener (2008) demonstrate that trusting and cooperative social relationships tended to enhance people's subjective wellbeing, and that, in turn, positive feelings of wellbeing tended to augment trust and cooperation. This bidirectional relationship was supported by empirical research. Tov and Diener assert that "[e]xtensive empirical work now supports the fact that sociability, interpersonal warmth, community involvement, and interpersonal trust are heightened by positive emotions" (2008, p. 155).

School-level and individual wellbeing are significantly enhanced through the power of positive relationships. Noble and McGrath (2008) write that, "positive peer relationships and positive teacher-pupil relationships help pupils to feel connected to school and to experience support and acceptance" (p. 122). There are many ways that we can encourage positive relationships and connectedness at work and in our lives. Marks (2011) proposes that building connections supports and enriches life, and that we can pay attention to the different kind of connections we have with others, thick and thin. He describes "[o]ur thick relationships [as] our close intimate relationships and our thin ones [as] our broader circle of friends, relatives work colleagues, neighbours and people we know in our daily lives" (Marks, 2011, pp. 4687–4691). Both types of relationships are vital for nourishing wellbeing.

Establishing and maintaining positive relationships with family, neighbors, colleagues, and friends, such that we meaningfully connect, contribute to, and benefit from the presence of other others in our lives, helps our social wellbeing. We've learned a great deal from Tom Rath's writings and the work from Gallup. From our reading of *Vital Friends* (Rath, 2006), we learned that, "strong social relationships are *the* leading indicator of our overall happiness, and these findings appear to hold up across countries and cultures" (p. 21). Rath (2006) maintains that "energy *between* two people is what creates great marriages, families, teams, and organizations" (p. 2). Indeed, friendships are among the most fundamental of human needs. Rath (2006) writes that, "As human beings, we want to take part in the same activities as our friends. Doing so makes us laugh and feel good, and it provides social support" (p. 56). Rath (2006) writes about the benefits and types of friendship that enhance all of life and suggests that friends are supports and "catalysts for high points in any given day" (p. 21). Whether it is sharing a long commute, working a tedious job, or determining a next move, a friend lifts our spirits, gives advice, and provides enjoyment. As one might guess, the dimension of wellbeing and friendship are connected to each other. For example, Rath (2006) states that, "If your best friend has a very healthy diet, you are five times as likely to have a very healthy diet yourself" (p. 24). So, the benefits of a kind friend to one's health are noted by researchers who have suggested that "[friendship] improves our cardiovascular functioning and resiliency and decreases our stress levels" (p. 25). In fact, having at least four friends helps people to live significantly longer. Rath (2006) writes that, "Over a four year span, people in the 'isolated' group (those with fewer than four friends) were *more than twice as likely to die* from heart disease" (p. 25). Rath (2006) asserts that "the absence of high-quality friendships is bad for our health, spirits, productivity, and longevity" (p. 26).

Researchers indicate that employers create positive or negative moods by the way they treat their employees which, in turn, will impact upon workers' work and family life. Rath (2006) found that "only 18% of people work for organizations that provide opportunities to develop friendships on the job" (p. 50). However, company loyalty was enhanced when employers recognized and affirmed that people want to forge quality friendships. According to Rath (2006), a vital friend is "someone who measurably improves your life; [and] a person at work or in your personal life whom you can't afford to live without" (p. 76). Rath and colleagues developed a measurement for eight of the most common friendship roles. *Builders* are catalysts for one's personal and professional growth: "[T]hese are the friends who lead you to achieve more each day" (Rath, 2006, p. 87). *Champions* act as advocates and loyal friends who thrive on others' happiness and accomplishments: "Champions stand up for you and what you believe in. They are the friends who sing your praises" (Rath, 2006, p. 93). *Collaborators* share interests, ambitions, and passions which provide a strong foundation for long-lasting friendships; someone with whom "You might share a passion for sports, hobbies, religion, work, politics, food, music, movies, or books" (Rath, 2006, p. 99). *Companions* are lifelong friends who share an unbreakable bond and will readily sacrifice for the other's benefit. Marriage partners may be considered Companions: "At times, a true Companion will even sense where you are headed—your thoughts, feelings, and actions—before you know it yourself" (Rath, 2006, p. 105). *Connectors* are acquainted with a large network of people and are helpful in introducing one to important others: "This [person] extends your network dramatically and gives you access to newfound resources" (Rath, 2006, p. 111). *Connectors* thrive in helping to establish links for people. *Energizers* are "fun friends" who bring laughter, smiles, and positivity into the day: "They are always saying and doing things that make you feel better" (Rath, 2006, p. 117). *Mind Openers* broaden one's perspective and challenge one to think in innovative ways: "Mind Openers are the friends who expand your horizons and encourage you to embrace new ideas, opportunities, cultures, and people" (Rath, 2006, p. 123). They ask questions that make their friends receptive to new ideas. *Navigators* give guidance, direction, and advice as one moves forward in life: "Any time you're at a crossroads and need help making a decision, you can look to a Navigator" (Rath, 2006, p. 129). Navigators are good listeners, can help determine the positive and negative aspects of a decision, and know the personality of the friend.

DEVELOPING A POSITIVE RELATIONSHIP TO THE BODY

The primacy of the body in regards to wellbeing was developed in chapter 2. Here we describe how the body is a different field of learning from which we can gather a different and more visceral understanding of our selves and our lives. Sight is often a privileged sense, foundational to our whole interpreted perspective. However, when we step back and out of our routine habits of being, we notice that much of human experience happens outside of the languaged realm of sight perspective. Attunement to the body is another practice that supports mindful alignment. Attuning to the body means engaging in practices in ways that acknowledge and honor the physical needs, sensations, intuitions, and emotions that are central to the human experience. Attuning to the body is an opportunity to live more fully, accessing multiple pathways to know and to be. Noticing embodied experiences means accessing what is going on right now in my body, for better or for worse, and this is an act of mindfulness. Rechtshchaffen (2014), a mindfulness educator and coach, explained that we all need to learn the language of our bodies since the sensations of the body are foundational to a rich relationship to our mind and our hearts. As one of our research participants shared, physical attunement opened them up to others in rewarding and sometimes unexpected ways:

> All of a sudden, little Davie got up and put his arms around me, and hugged me. He had never done that all year, and then he sat down again and continued his craft. And then he said a few minutes later in a very loud voice, "This is the best day of my life." And it moved me to tears because we were just doing a simple craft at center time and this little guy, he was feeling so good about himself, that he had just gotten to a point where everyone could accept him.

Examples of powerful emotional responses, such as being moved to tears by attuning to the emotions of others, were commonly described when educators looked for ways to account for their own flourishing. Equally expressed were sensations of pride, amazement, and awe. Interesting that these experiences were re-experienced through the body as they are recalled, evidenced in the joy and smiling and earnest engagement of the participants telling their stories. Interesting how simply hearing the stories of others can give us such a sense of physical energy and warmth of heart.

How we come to know the world around us is called "epistemology," or ways of knowing. Different cultures embrace different epistemological assumptions. Inoue (2012) describes how a Japanese understanding of epistemology includes the awareness that most of our personal theories stem from "gut feelings." The Japanese term for this is *jikkan*. While experiencing gut feelings and sensations may be a common human experience, different cultures give different value and voice to these intuitions. Inoue (2012) suggests that cultures that under-explore knowledge created in, with, and from the body would greatly benefit from greater investigation into gut responses. As part of our interest in mindful awareness as a professional learning opportunity for educators, we see the importance of paying attention to the body as a site for learning.

While it may seem like bodily responses are spontaneous, they can also be intentionally fostered. First, we can learn to pay attention to the body to notice and interpret sensations and signals from and in the body as learning opportunities. Second, we can create environmental supports and structures for attuning to the body as a site for rich and important learning. For example, from our research we noticed that the experiences of attuning to the body and creating deeper connections with others were often enhanced by food; we recognize that sharing meals is a habit of creating and sustaining community across cultures, as communal eating opportunities can nourish us on physical, mental, emotional, and spiritual levels. As one participant aptly explained, "It is all about the food. Someone would always bring food into the staff room and I think food is the connecting aspect, that breaking bread concept. I think that it's really important in those down times." Others described the fun and spontaneous laughter that opportunities to sit together over food brought to her staff: "Every time we are sitting around this table in our staff room, we are laughing. Our whole lunch hour is laughter—constant, constant laughter, and that feels good." As we explore more deeply the relationship between mindfulness and noticing what feels good, we become more fully appreciative of the wisdom from Thich Nhat Hanh (n.d.), the great Zen master, who famously explained to talk show host Oprah the practice of what has come to be know as the tea meditation:

> If you are ruminating about the past, or worrying about the future, you will completely miss the experience of enjoying the cup of tea. You will look down at the cup, and the tea will be gone. Life is like that. If you are not fully present, you will look around and it will be gone. You will have missed the feel, the aroma, the delicacy and beauty of life.

Nhat Hanh says that "mindfulness allows us to live" (1975, p. 15). It is how we continually restore ourselves, and is a simple, but powerful practice that can attune us to the aliveness in simple moments. This simplicity is mindfulness and, as Ragoonaden (2015) describes it, this involves "abandoning the lure of complexity to embrace the dynamic simplicity of being present" (p. 17). As we pay attention to our body as a site of learning, we can metaphorically and literally attend to our tea—there is no haste—to notice how the moment is alive in the body and appreciated in the mind, body, and spirit.

As we have been describing, the physical experience of wellbeing is part and parcel of the emotional experience—as we attune to our bodies, we start to notice and attune to the stories that live in our bodies. These stories can provide a deep sense of learning about how we are engaging life in authentic ways. We can also cultivate learning through attending more closely to our physical sensations and actions, such as by smiling or by creating connections such as handshakes and hugs. As we will describe, engaging in the physical act of listening from a mindful approach of paying deep attention is a wonderful opportunity for creating and sustaining connections with others. Part of healthy and happy relationships is being an active and empathic listener, being present with and recognizing the other. Ben-Shahar (2012) noted that when one chooses to listen "to provide the space and the opportunity for others to share experiences, feelings, and thoughts" (p. 69), the other feels heard and recognized. As educators, we can choose to actively engage in seeing, listening, and appreciating each person as a worthy and valuable human being, being fully present to them in ways that reflect back to them who they are and who they can continue to become through ongoing love, learning, and growth.

DEVELOPING A MINDFUL APPROACH TO LISTENING

In your experience, how high on the list of personal attributes possessed by the best of friends would you find the quality of being a "good listener"? Our experience suggests that "excellent listener" is one of the most commonly cited features of a friend. As we have been described, listening is an act of reciprocity or mutual exchange within a relationship. When carried out as a mindful act of caring for the other, listening can become a gateway to building compassion and love. Awareness of how we listen is the starting point to developing a loving approach to the relational nature of our lives. Martin Buber, the twentieth-century social philosopher, helps explain the difference between surface listening and genuine, affirming, and attentive listening. Basically, Buber maintains that there are two primal relationships: *I–Thou* and *I–It*. Within the I–It relationship, we respond to others as objects ("It"s) whom we manipulate to fulfill our own purposes. In seeing others as objects, we (I) ourselves are not authentic but rather respond in ways that try to control or manipulate the other. We listen to satisfy our purposes with little regard for the other. The alternative, rarer, and more "connecting" way is the I–Thou relationship in which one abandons the objectifying outlook and manipulation and enters into an authentic relationship. Buber's idea was to embrace the other in dialogue, where the relationship is of primary importance. The listener offers herself or himself, authentically and honestly, to the speaker. The aim is not pragmatic or for usefulness but, rather, to understand the other person and to be understood by her or him. Buber believes that when the I–Thou relationship is exercised, individual worth is experienced through the deep human connection. Gordon (2011) asserts, "This encountering the other, this embracing of the other refers, to the act of identifying with someone's position and lived situation while simultaneously maintain a clear sense of self" (p. 212). Genuine listening is to open up, loving with acceptance of the other, in order to understand the full dimension of what the individual is trying to express.

Listening with a deep presence, awareness, and from a stance of love and care toward the other can cultivate moments of understanding or sensing what another is feeling or going through. This empathy is an important starting point for compassion, which can be understood as the desire to alleviate the suffering of another (Worline & Dutton, 2017). While not often assumed to be part of the work in organizations, compassion researchers are starting to understand the power and potential of compassion as a necessary ingredient in successful organizations of all kinds. As we found with the educators in our research, when they work in a school where they know others care about them and they care about their colleagues, this tends to increase and improve their commitment, engagement, and enjoyment of their work. Indeed, compassion research bears out the fact that organizations that value and support compassion in the workplace tend to report greater levels of employee engagement, commitment, and quality of work (Worline & Dutton, 2017).

We recently read a beautiful book detailing a week-long conversation between two exemplars of compassion and love, his Holiness the Dalai Llama and Archbishop Desmond Tutu (Abrams, 2016). These two men described the important role that compassion has played in cultivating their sense of joy, despite lives filled with enormous hardship. They shared how the choice to remain open-hearted and searching for the good in all humans is available to each of us, but that we need to engage in regular practices to develop and sustain this compassionate approach to life. The Dalai Llama and the Archbishop Tutu exemplify what it means to have a "mind-set toward shared humanity" (Woreline & Dutton, 2017, p. 51), and they have demonstrated the power of living from a relational belief, knowing that we are all interconnected and part of the same human story. In the book, Tutu shared his culture's beliefs about Ubuntu, an African philosophy that recognizes that each of us are connected and beholden to the other in a tapestry of humanity, that "I am me because of you." This idea of engaging with others with a sense of deep interconnectedness and love is reflected in many other world religions and philosophies, such as the Christian rule to "treat others as you would have them treat you," or the Hindu and Buddhist ideas of Karma and reincarnation where we reap in the next life what we sow in this life. As we will describe, deep and attentive listening with an attunement to holding the other as "thou," within a space of love and compassion, can be a transformative practice for each person in the listening relationship.

THE ART OF LISTENING

There are various reasons to listen, and we propose that listening can be a gateway to more care, compassion, and love. Of course, listening to one another is also critical to success in business, informative and therapeutic in health care and training, foundational to understanding and learning for students and staff in education, and listening enhances and strengthens family and social life. As we listen, we share in the joy as others express elation of celebratory events, and we walk beside those who unload burdens. Some listen to those who seek spiritual direction or require help in clarifying goals. Others listen to attain knowledge and information. Listening supports professional and personal life; the elements of recognition, attention, affirmation, care, and encouragement are part of good listening practice.

The type of listening we will focus on is *interpersonal listening*, as a way of thinking about how we can foster and sustain meaningful, positive relationships at work. Scholars use different terminology to describe interpersonal listening but the focus is on the "other" or the speaker. Milton (2000) terms this "friendly listening or benevolent listening" (p. 52), highlighting one's attentive and nonjudgmental attitude toward the other. Other researchers term effective listening *empathic* or *active listening*, where it is defined as "an attempt to demonstrate unconditional acceptance and unbiased reflection [of the speaker] . . . without the listener's own interpretive structures intruding on his or her understanding of the other person" (Weger, Castle, & Emmett, 2010, p. 35).

What Does Listening Mean?

Etymologically, the word *listen* comes from a Gothic root that emphasized attention to another (*Online Etymology Dictionary*). The International Listening Association defined listening as "the process of receiving, constructing meaning from, and responding to spoken and/or non-verbal messages" (online at www.listen.org). Jones (2011) defines listening in a similar way: "the ability to effectively attend to, interpret, and respond to verbal and nonverbal messages" (p. 86). She explains that listening is a multidimensional construct that consists of cognitive processes such as understanding, receiving, and interpreting to the messages. Listening also employs affective processes such as being motivated to attend to the other and behavioral processes such as responding with verbal and nonverbal strategies (p. 85).

Why is Listening Especially Important for Educators?

In contemporary society, isolation, stress, worry, and a general sense of unwellness are experienced by many people. Milton (2000) notes that, "A growing number of people now find themselves troubled by feelings of solitude, both physical and spiritual, and this is affecting people well beyond any marginalized sectors of society" (p. 52). People from all walks of life need to be affirmed, understood, and cared for, elements which are part of "friendly," "benevolent," "empathic," or "active" listening.

Listening enables colleagues to work better together, and Mineyama et al. (2007) found that when supervisors listened with empathy and unconditional positive regard, and practiced specific listening skills and techniques, subordinates perceived that they were cared for and there was a reduction of psychological stress (p. 86). In the field of nursing, patients who perceived they were listened to expressed contentment and peace. Shipley (2010) affirms: "The therapeutic use of listening may contribute to the patient's over-all sense of wellbeing and satisfaction with the healthcare experience" (p. 126).

Indeed, everyone needs to be understood by someone who is significant to them. Kagan (cited in Shipley, 2010) reports that "people desire to be listened to more than anything else during their experiences with health professionals" (p. 126). Also, listening contributes to the self and personality development field (Pasupathi & Billitteri, 2015). Pasupathi and Billitteri (2015) write, "A good listening to . . . matters a great deal for influencing people's sense of themselves" (p. 68). They say a superb listener can allow "the speaker to hear his or her own internal conflicts and dialogue more clearly" (Pasupathi & Billitteri, 2015, p. 79). To recognize the importance of listening may lead to improving the lives and wellness of those who work and live together.

As we listen to our colleagues, we may notice a deeper sense of connection and empathy, of understanding them and their situations. Worline and Dutton (2017) suggest that the act of noticing the suffering of others is the portal, or gateway, to "awakening compassion at work" (p. 33). We see how listening from a mindset of shared humanity—knowing that the person in front of me is worthy of my time and care because we are interconnected in this shared humanity—can be a subtle but powerful shift toward a relational approach with our colleagues. The resulting contribution of developing a relational approach through deep listening based in love, respect, care, and compassion is that flourishing at work can take place. We recall a recent example of the power of mindful listening for the purpose of expressing loving-kindness at a recent mindfulness class for teachers. In this session, we paired up and were instructed to take turns sharing whatever came to mind about our experiences of mindfulness so far that day. The listener was to be fully present and share loving-kindness as their only task. At the end of this experience of giving and receiving mindful listening, we were motivated to share and duplicate this experience with our friends, families, and colleagues at work. Taking the time to give and receive love, peace, acceptance, or compassion was a tremendously uplifting and energizing experience for both people in the listening relationship.

MINDFUL ART PRACTICE FOR POSITIVE RELATIONSHIPS: DEEP LISTENING

The key elements to enhance listening include empathy, silence, attention to both verbal and non-verbal communication, and the ability to be nonjudg-mental and accepting. In addition, listening is an explicit and deliberate act that recognizes and commits to the other. Listening is a skill that may be taught and should be encouraged (Mineyama et al., 2007; Weger, Castle, & Emmett, 2010).

Empathy

Empathy, the crucial element for listening, occurs when one becomes aware of, and identifies with the thoughts, experiences, and feelings of another (Merriam-Webster Online Dictionary). Pence and James (2015) note that "good listening implies empathic, person-centered listening" (p. 85). Some positive outcomes when empathy is practiced "[include] helping the support-seeker cope with emotional stress and increase in . . . life satisfaction" (p. 86). Empathy enables the speaker to feel safe and accepted while sharpening the listener's ability to understand. Shipley (2010) maintains that "[t]he use of empathy conveys to the speaker that the listener is fully present and actively engaged in the encounter" (p. 130). Brownell (2013) described an empathetic listener as one who

> strives to thoroughly and accurately understand the person speaking; he does not direct the conversation, but [rather] encourages the other person to share his ideas and feelings. The empathic listener does not impose his own opinions or values. When listening empathically, you don't evaluate; rather, you promote honest, engaged communication through total other-centered involvement in the encounter. (p. 174)

An interesting finding was that females demonstrate a significantly greater ability to respond in an active-empathic manner (Pence & James, 2014, p. 92).

Verbal and Nonverbal Communication

Listening effectively incorporates both verbal and nonverbal communication where the listener gains deep understanding by observing tone of voice, body language, and considers a person's cultural background. Shipley (2010) notes, "The listener . . . constantly strives to understand the spoken message as well as perceive the underlying meanings and ones of the encounter" (p. 133). Much may be understood and interpreted through nonverbal communication as Brownell (2013) noted: "Studies conducted in the United States indicate that nonverbal factors carry more than 65 percent of the meaning of an interpersonal message" (p. 181). Bodie et al. (2012) found that listening competence included "responsiveness, eye contact, questioning, understanding, conversational flow and [being] friendly or polite" (p. 7). Understanding one's culture may also influence understanding in listening. Brownell (2013) states that "the Swiss, German, and Scandinavian cultures tend to be . . . more explicit and direct in their verbal messages" (p. 184).

Attending to the Listener

Once the speaker chooses to share with the listener, the subsequent shaping of the sharing is an interactive dyadic process with mutual contributions. Pasupathi and Billiteri (2015) note that when listeners incorporate unintrusive yet attentive body language, "attentive listeners are actively co-constructing the narrative with the narrator" (p. 72). Though the listener does not interrupt, it is important he offer signals of attentiveness and comprehension using "physical gestures and brief auditory responses such as 'mm-mmm' and 'yeah' often termed 'backchannels'" (Pasupathi & Billiteri, 2015, p. 72). Jones (2011) also asserts that supportive listening requires the listener to "demonstrate emotional involvement and attunement while attending to, interpreting, and responding to the emotions of the support seeker; a complex and challenging task" (p. 86). Brownell (2013) includes a list of warm behaviors that welcome and encourage the speaker, including direct eye contact, touching, smiling, nodding, eyes wide open, forward lean, and positive facial expression (p. 189). On the contrary, if listeners are perceived to be inactive, the speaker may assume disinterest and forego deep sharing but rather share "events and perceptions as less typical of themselves" (Pasupathi & Billiteri, 2015, p. 73). The attentive listener self-monitors and consciously attends to the speaker.

Trust and Safety

We focused on the importance of trust earlier, but we need to remind our readers that the development of trust within a listening relationship allows for authentic sharing and greater risk-taking. Hart (1980) states, "It is the choice to welcome another warmly and to provide an environment in which the other can feel safe. It is a choice to listen to another with attention and interest, to affirm and confirm all that one can" (p. 19). Also, it is critical to keep confidences. Petersen (2007) states, "When we really listen, we don't use information shared in trust against talkers or others, then, or at a later time" (p. 94). Indeed, the purpose of active listening is to demonstrate understanding without judgment. Weger, Castle, and Emmett (2010) assert that "[a]n active listening response builds empathy and trust with the speaker by showing unconditional regard for him/her and confirming his/her experience" (p. 36).

Nonjudgmental Listening

When one is listening attentively, Milton (2000) advocates "this type of listening is based on not judging others but focuses on the person you are listening to" (p. 52). To establish a culture of safety and the freedom to truly share concerns, the elements of respect, acceptance, and trust are paramount.

To understand what the speaker is communicating, it is helpful to suspend one's own biases and preferences. Shipley (2010) reminds listeners to understand "the whole person and [recognize] that each person is a unique individual with different beliefs, lifestyles, and cultures" (p. 130). Respect for the other, recognition of their uniqueness and autonomy, and the presumption of good will are elements of nonjudgmental listening.

To Clarify

Listening to speakers helps them to recognize and develop their thoughts and to determine their actions. Good listeners understand that they do not "own the problem" (Petersen, 2007, p. 75), because each experience is unique and belongs to the speaker. The listener expresses respect, care, and concern, realizing that "listening is a more effective and empowering way to help others than trying to solve their problems for them" (Petersen, 2007, p. 75). Also, the speaker is seldom helped by the listener providing an analogy or similar story of something he or she has experienced or by sharing solutions. Rather, the listener provides understanding, clarification, and encouragement as the speaker takes charge of his or her life.

To be Deliberate

Listening is a deliberate act and requires one to be fully present. Brownell (2013) affirms that "listening takes time . . . you need to choose to listen" (p. 5). In the profession of nursing, Shipley (2010) states, "For effective listening to occur, the nurse must make a conscious decision to be fully present and engaged in the patient encounter" (p. 130). Indeed, listening demands being fully present and attentive where one's needs and concerns are set aside. To listen in a meaningful way, the valuable elements of time commitment and mental energy are necessary. Fatigue, a busy schedule, and personal concerns are realities that need to be addressed. Jones (2011) reports that the one seeking assistance or requesting support "is often viewed as relationally burdensome and face-threatening" (p. 88). It takes time, courage, and patience to provide supportive listening to others.

To be a Companion

The willingness of an educator to enter into a supportive relationship is to be a companion where one agrees to go alongside. To be a savior, a teacher, or one with advice may run contrary to this purpose. If the listener is too talkative, asks too many questions, or shares personal stories, the speaker may feel less free to share deeply and authentically. In addition, it is less helpful if the listener is too directive and controlling in advice. Indeed, Jones (2011) reports research indicating "that advice is often neither well received nor wanted in the first place" (p. 90). Rather, what is preferred is the listener being emotionally connected and centered on the speaker whereby the speaker reports "feeling better" (Jones, 2011, p. 87).

To Provide Emotional Support

By providing emotional support to the one experiencing difficulties, his or her ability to cope may be strengthened which would lead to an improvement in wellbeing. Being present and focused on the speaker, Jones (2011) highlights, "validates the difficult emotional experiences of the distressed person by explicitly acknowledging them in talk" (p. 87). The listener is encouraged to name the emotions expressed by the speaker. Jones further highlights the importance of "psychological and physiological closeness, warmth and openness to engage" (p. 87) as elements of support. The supportive listener pays attention to the emotional cues of the speaker.

Silence

When the listener is silent, this allows the speaker time and the freedom to communicate without interruption. Though extended silence may feel uncomfortable, it may encourage the speaker to go deeper. Ferrari (2012) writes, "If you succeed in keeping still and quiet, you might create a moment or two of uncomfortable silence. Don't be afraid of that . . . you could be very surprised by what insightful comment your CPs blurt out during these lulls" (p. 46). Also, good listeners do not interrupt the speaker but allow him or her to express the essential concerns that may remain hidden and unspoken if interrupted.

Paraphrasing and Questioning

Speakers may feel that they are heard and understood when the listener reflects, paraphrases, and gives feedback on what was communicated. Researchers have shown that if a speaker perceives that the listener to be distracted, the speaker may view him or her "not only unresponsive, but also as disagreeing with their narrative" (Pasupathi & Billiteri, 2015, p. 74). Rather, research indicates a positive outcome from paraphrasing may be an increase in likeability (Weger, Castle, & Emmett, 2010). Weger, Castle, and Emmett (2010) state, "Listeners who paraphrase a speaker's message communicate interest in, and perhaps tacit endorsement of, the speaker's message and perhaps create a greater sense of closeness or immediacy" (p. 44). People "tend to disclose more information to those they initially like than to people whom they dislike" (Weger, Castle, & Emmett, 2010, p. 45).

When paraphrasing, the atmosphere of calmness, safety, and understanding may be enhanced. Pattersen et al. (2012) encourage listeners to not just parrot back what was said, but to "put the message in your own words—usually in an abbreviated form" (p. 89). When skillfully done, posing questions that elicit additional information in a speaker's narrative will provide elaborations of ideas and thoughts and can provide needed insights into the speaker's sense of wellbeing. Worline and Dutton (2017) describe the work of listening and posing questions designed to draw out the speaker's hidden suffering as the inquiry work of noticing that is needed for compassionate acting (p. 35). Suffering is a hindrance to commitment, engagement, and quality of work, and is also hurtful to our shared humanity. However, sharing our suffering at work is not always valued or accepted and can often be hidden by fear, embarrassment, and shame. Even in organizational settings that value and promote compassionate acting at work, suffering can be felt as "inexpressibility, meaning that the experience of suffering and what it means to us are almost impossible to adequately convey to others" (Worline & Dutton, 2017, p. 37). Compassionate colleagues can notice and do the gentle probing needed to allow the suffering to surface, and hopefully provide alleviation of that suffering.

Within the medical field, Jones (2011) highlights the importance of shared understanding reached when "both doctor and patient actively listen to one another by asking questions and paraphrasing what was said" (p. 89). Questions are for clarification and to receive additional information. Brownell (2013) says that probing questions are helpful "when you don't feel you are getting adequate information to understand your partner's point of view thoroughly" (p. 113). To paraphrase and question the speaker will indicate attentiveness and concern.

In this chapter, we have described how our sense of wellbeing includes attending to positive relationships with our emotions, with others, and with our selves, through attending to our body as a site of learning. We suggest that positive relationships are strengthened through careful listening. Developing the art of a mindful approach to listening can happen through practices of empathy, nonjudgment, and silence (to name a few). In the next chapter, we describe the role of recognizing personal strengths and values in developing mindful awareness. We also describe how appreciation and self-compassion are supported through the mindful art of meditative letter writing.

Chapter Four

Higher Purpose in Work and Strength-Based Living

Through our research, we have become fascinated with the notion that, if we shift the lens we use to view the world through paying attention to what helps us flourish, our lives and the lives of others can be transformed. We suggest that this attention to what helps us and others to flourish will provide profound insights into one's professional learning journey. This attention to flourishing means attending to how we express our truest and our most authentic selves in the context of our work as educators. Imagine a school where the educators, students, staff, and all others in the learning community engage as leaders of learning toward actualizing for themselves and others what it means to flourish. Imagine a whole community of learners seeking to discover what it means to move forward in ways that authentically fill out each of their highest potentials. As we have shared, at the heart of this book is the idea that we can shift our experiences through the poetic and Pygmalion principles which remind us that, by shifting the questions we ask, the expectations that we hold, and by paying attention to the stories that shape and influence our social realities, we can make this powerful workplace learning imaginable. Of course, we do so in ways that align with our most deeply held values and our core, life affirming, beliefs.

In his extensive writing about what it means to be an authentic, thoughtful, and effective teacher, Parker Palmer (1998; 1999a; 1999b; 2004) suggests that teachers need to know themselves as part of the process of engaging in healthy, growth-oriented relationships with students. We agree, and suggest that knowing oneself is essential to reclaiming a sense of self-cultivation as part of the work of teaching—that teachers can, and should, model for their students what it means to grow and learn as a human through their work as educators (Higgins, 2011; Starratt, 2004).

For most educators, professional learning is an ongoing responsibility for continuing to improve our practice in the service of improving students' learning experiences. For many of us, professional learning has been experienced as a set of focused strategies for fixing or repairing aspects of our practice that we, or others, perceive to be deficient or broken. We attend workshops or read books or connect with other educators in learning conversations designed to find, address, and fix the problems we see in ourselves, in others, and in the system. How many of us have experienced a Thursday or Friday "workshop high" which has prompted us to aspire to make transformative change, but found that the enthusiasm and laudable intentions have been displaced on Monday by forgetfulness, a rationalized sense of contentment (inertia), or the survival routines that help us to cope? This is a sad, vicious cycle, experienced time and again by many educator colleagues. This idea of focusing on fixing what is wrong or on ways of overcoming perceived deficiencies is a common way of thinking about personal, professional, or organizational improvement. Aligned with our premise that what we pay attention to grows, we offer an alternative perspective to this traditional approach to change for improvement. We suggest that if we want to feel a sense of wellbeing in our work—of feeling engaged, connected, on purpose, and alive in our work, in service of encouraging others to experience the same—that we can find more of this as we shift the lens of improvement toward flourishing through using an appreciative and compassionate approach to working with self and others.

We see the process of recalibrating, or attuning, to our strengths, values, goals, and desires as an important shift in professional development, one that leads us toward cultivating a sense of meaning and purpose in our work. While we are realistic and know that there are many aspects of ourselves that are likely in need of improvement, we believe that a focus on what we most hope to grow is likely to give us more of what we want, rather than focusing on what is not working and noticing merely what is missing as a result. From this appreciative perspective, then, coming to know oneself is about noticing and nurturing strengths, talents, virtues, and values, and then creating opportunities to live these out at work. Each of us is unique and brings different character traits, talents, interests, and resources to our work. We build strength through use and practice. And so it makes sense that we might begin to identify those traits, interests, and talents that we most frequently express because they come most naturally to us, or we enjoy using them, or the use of them makes us feel positive in some way. Understanding our various strengths can give us clues to how we can craft our work and lives to feel more engaged, happier, and more productive.

Character strengths can be described as values and virtues inherent in all humans that make up our positive identity. These have been highlighted through ancient wisdom and traditions as the capacities that make us human and that help build up healthy individuals and communities—courage, humility, honor, gratitude, and trustworthiness. Based on research findings on the generative potential of positive practices to enhance wellbeing, Park, Petersen, and Seligman (2004) established a set of twenty-four character strengths—personal values and virtues—that resonate across all cultures. These researchers then set out to study whether living from these personal strengths enhanced and increased happiness and overall wellbeing. These twenty-four character strengths are available to everyone, at all times, and the researchers suggest that becoming aware of our strengths and then finding ways to consciously express our highest strengths in an intentional and sustained way leads to improvement in all aspects of our lives. These strengths are organized by virtues that are appreciated and cultivated across all cultures (wisdom, courage, humanity, justice, temperance, and transcendence). Within each of these sets of virtues are values that are understood as strengths. For example, the appreciation of beauty and excellence, or gratitude, are strengths within the virtue of transcendence. Love of learning and curiosity are the strengths in the virtue of wisdom.

While each of us has the potential to express each of the twenty-four strengths, signature strengths, a smaller set of strengths that we tend to use most often in our daily lives, tend to reflect our unique personality. Studies have shown that as we learn to actively cultivate our signature character strengths we can improve our satisfaction and happiness, whether at work or in life (Hodges & Asplund, 2010; Young, Kashdon, & Macatee, 2014). These researchers suggest that as we use our particular set of traits, we will be expressing our best and most authentic sense of self. From a more pragmatic view, living from these signature character strengths provides the substance, fuel, or energy needed for building other talents or pursuing other interests. For example, imagine you want to build stronger relationships at work to be able to collaborate more significantly with your colleagues. You might choose to use your signature strengths of curiosity and perseverance in pursuit of this goal. Using curiosity to fuel a learning adventure about collaboration as well as a learning adventure about your colleagues, and perseverance will come in handy to stay the course when relationships are slow to build or when sought-after collaboration goes sideways. The intentional use of these strengths provides an opportunity to frame an existing challenge in new ways, such as could be useful for engaging curiosity in an existing relationship to come to know a colleague in a new light. Using your particular strength of curiosity feels good to you and creates a positive benefit in your own work. This is not to say that we should only work from a small set of strengths, but that we can learn to use our signature strengths more often as we build up our middle strengths and those strengths that rarely show up in our lives as part of the ongoing work of filling out our lives in balanced ways.

As with all things human, there is a potential flip side to using our strengths in ways that leads to improvement and enrichment of self and other. For example, overusing honesty can lead to being too blunt, overplaying humor can lead to telling jokes at the wrong time, or overplaying zest can lead to exhaustion. Finding a middle ground where you learn about the best use of your strengths, all of them, in pursuit of filling out your potentials in ways that contributes to a common good is the path toward more engagement, meaning and purpose in work and life (Hodges & Asplund, 2010; Young, Kashdon, & Macatee, 2014). All of these strengths will shift and change over time, and so knowing who we are, what we hold important and how we choose to live our strengths at work requires ongoing reflection and personal assessment.

The art of coming to know personal strengths and values can happen in an appreciative way as we access moments in our lives where we feel aligned, where our actions seem to be in tune with our values, and where we are using our strengths in ways that help us connect and contribute in our work and our life. Engaging from a strengths-based perspectives has been shown to increase happiness, connection, commitment, and a sense of being able to do more and be more in other areas of our lives (Achor, 2011; Fredrickson & Losada, 2005; Park, Petersen, & Seligman, 2004). One of the educators in our research shared the importance of helping the students to understand that we need to spend time getting to know the strengths and values that are present in each of us in a group in order to work well together. He described:

> One of the activities I do at the beginning of the year is I get all the kids outside and I put them into groups and I get them to make a human pyramid. They can get down on their hands and knees and they can get up onto each other's backs and they can see how high they can get. And always, the pyramids fall down. But they have to learn to work together and they don't know why I am doing that at the beginning, but they try hard and they work together. When we are back in the classroom, I tell them that that pyramid is like our classroom. We need to work together to make that pyramid work. If we were to take one brick out of that pyramid whether it is the bottom brick or whatever, the whole thing starts to collapse and I say we are all very important bricks in this pyramid and if we start to get after one person or nag one person or leave one person out, then it starts to hurt our whole classroom and we need to work together to make our pyramid strong.

This educator recognized the importance of providing a practice for the students to understand how to appreciate all the different pieces of their group as a whole, to help each other support each other to work well together. We have seen how appreciation can be a powerful tool for cultivating more balanced environments in our schools, where teachers are working with students to promote more than just increased test scores, they are co-creating generative, life-giving systems of learning.

Organizations are places where people interact for a variety of intended outcomes. Although organizations start out as the relationships among and between people, "over time they become separated from people, functioning in pursuit of their own goals and purposes. This separation has to be bridged somehow" (Sergiovanni & Starratt, 1993, p. 6). What would we notice in our organizations if we embraced and celebrated the complexities and challenges that our membership in them brings, rather than perceiving them as something that needs to be fixed? Shifting our focus to pay attention to that which we wish to grow is at the heart of appreciative processes for transformational change, where we can always notice something that works. When we remember that what we focus on becomes our reality, we can choose to find and then reflect on what works well, to appreciate the present moment knowing that it is one reality among many possibilities that we can co-construct with others (Coghlan, Preskill, & Tzavaras Catsambas, 2003; Whitney & Trosten-Bloom, 2010).

PAYING ATTENTION TO THOUGHTS

As described in the introduction, Victor Frankl's logotherapy philosophy has influenced millions of people across many contexts and provides important insights on how learning to attune to our strengths, values, and intentions is a powerful way to cultivate ourselves in our work in every moment. Predicated on the belief that we each have agency in every moment to choose our response to any situation, Frankl resolves that finding meaning in our experiences through how we think about them is a key ingredient to constructing a meaningful life. He argues that this can happen as we engage with awareness in the present moment. He believes that "when we stay true to our personal values in our professional lives, we lay a foundation of meaning. When we work in awareness of the moment, we stay connected to meaning. Our existence, and the existence of life, is meaning . . . by not being prisoners of our thoughts, and by not working against ourselves, we bring meaning to work" (as cited in Pattakos, 2010, p. 128). Frankl recognizes the power of our thoughts for transforming our reality if we remain aware of the present moment and stay open to the possibility of attuning with an appreciative perspective and with the premise of finding ways to learn from all our experiences.

This learning mindset is a key part of cultivating a sense of meaning in our work and is an important element of attending to our strengths, values, and intentions. One's mindset, or how one thinks, influences one's flourishing. What we believe about ourselves influences images of self, behavior, and how we think about the future. Carol Dweck's (2006) research on growth mindsets shows that "the view you adopt for yourself profoundly affects the way you lead your life" (p. 6). She advocated a *growth mindset* whereby, through challenge, effort, persistence, practice, and determination one may learn and succeed. Mindset is more important than talent and ability. Those who maintain that one's abilities and intelligence are fixed and permanent are in the fixed mindset. A growth mindset includes having a passion for learning, a determination to overcome deficiencies, a willingness to confront challenges, a desire to have friends and colleagues who challenge one to grow, and a willingness to seek out and engage in new and stretching experiences. The hallmark of the growth mindset, writes Dweck (2006), is to have "The passion for stretching yourself and sticking to it, even (or especially) when it's not going well" (p. 7). The growth mindset is based on the belief that one's basic qualities can be enhanced, strengthened, and developed through application and experience. Failure, for the growth mindset, is a painful experience but it does not define the learner leading to a desire to continue seeking other paths toward the desired outcome.

Certainly, words and actions from others are a big influence on how we think about ourselves. However, a powerful source of messages and thoughts that is within our control in terms of how we listen and how we learn to receive, and then ultimately how we learn to re-direct and craft differently these messages, is from ourselves. How we think about our abilities tends to result in matching performance; Achor (2011) describes that, "Beliefs are so powerful because they dictate our efforts and actions" (p. 77). As an example, we know from research, and from our practice as educators, that when we tell students that they are intelligent, this can result in higher performance. This is known as the *Pygmalion Effect*, "when our belief in another person's potential brings that potential to life" (Achor, 2011, p. 84). Nonverbal and verbal messages are transformed into reality. When we choose to see the potential in our students, or our colleagues and tell them so explicitly we can guide and direct their behaviors toward improved outcomes. As Ben-Shahar (2012) writes, research consistently shows that, "The expectations of others—be they teachers, parents, managers, or military commanders—significantly impact the performance of their students, employees, and soldiers. To a great extent, we get what we expect of others: Beliefs are self-fulfilling prophecies" (p. 234).

Our recognition of the importance of how thoughts can drive behavior is crucial. For adults whose aim it is to help students develop a growth mindset, Dweck (2006) encourages them to teach "children to love challenges, be intrigued by mistakes, enjoy effort, and keep on learning" (p. 177). Able educators praise children and youth for what they accomplish because of their choice to practice, to study, to persist, and to use good strategies. A praising statement may be something like, "you really studied for your test and your improvement shows it. You read the material over several times, you outlined, it, and you tested yourself on it. It really worked" (p. 177). Teachers with a growth mindset "believe in the growth of the intellect and talent, and they are fascinated with the process of learning," says Dweck (2006, p. 194). These educators believe all children and youth can learn; they teach them to practice and persevere through the hard tasks and to be disciplined and responsible. As teachers display a growth mindset and set high standards for all of their students, showing them genuine affection within a disciplined environment, students thrive. Within a challenging environment, students are taught to learn, to think for themselves and to continue to practice fundamentals. Teachers who believe that all children can learn expect them to put in the effort and the required work hard. If there is a gap in learning, Dweck writes, "Growth-minded teachers tell students the truth and then give them the tools to close the gap" (p. 199). They tell the student they will not give up on them and will show them the necessary learning strategies needed to accomplish their goals. Giving constructive criticism helps young persons to achieve their learning or living goals and helps them to learn ways of doing the task better.

Taking what we know from research on the importance of building a growth mindset, of learning to guide our thoughts in ways that encourages learning and building from mistakes, we can see how important it is to create the conditions (internal and external) for us to keep learning and growing. We have found that attuning to the stories—those we tell ourselves and those we hear from others—in ways that encourages us to notice and nurture an appreciative and compassionate perspective is a powerful strategy for cultivating conditions where educators can feel a sense of flourishing. With this flourishing intention, we can learn to shift our attention to that which is meaningful to us, as opposed to fixating on what might be seen as a problem, stressor or negative challenge. Finding ways to notice and nurture our higher values in our work and extending ourselves toward something greater than our own piece of existence leads to an overall sense of living a meaningful life (Pattakos, 2010).

PAYING ATTENTION TO PRESENCE AND SELF-COMPASSION

Gaining a sense of awareness in the moment and an ability to detach from the thoughts and stories that so easily tether us to our sense of frustration, disappointment, disillusionment and dissatisfaction can lead toward building moments of meaning in our lives. We are not suggesting that we engage in the denial of suffering and difficulty, but we follow Frankl's advice that "if one cannot change a situation that causes his suffering, he can still choose his attitude" (p. 172) and that this is possible with the distinctly human ability of perspective-taking to notice an alternate possible response that enables us to see that meaning is always present in each moment (Frankl, 1984). We need to practice becoming present and fully aware of the moment, learn to notice and detach from stories and thoughts so that we can choose an attitude that leads toward fulfillment of our values and goals.

From a psychological perspective, coming to an awareness of the thoughts and stories that do limit our thinking and keep us entrenched in repeating negative or stifling behaviors can be a way out of what has been called the self-improvement trap (Flowers & Stahl, 2011, p. 95). This trap happens as we fail to notice the inherent worthiness of each of us and work instead to relentlessly work repair the deficiencies we see in ourselves. We tend to do this as we listen and internalize the negative messages from our environments. In turn, we interpret these messages to mean that we are separate from everybody else and that we are not enough or sufficient as we are. This deficit trap is a common one and has been felt by everyone at some point in their lives. Flowers and Stahl (2011) suggest that we can stay in the self-improvement trap for many years before we come to an awareness of the violence that we do to ourselves and to others as we endlessly strive for a false sense of perfection that we believe will, once attained, provide us with the merits for feeling a true sense of worthiness. This fallacy in our thinking keeps us in a personal prison built by our thoughts (Pattakos, 2010).

Flowers and Stahl (2011) suggest that the way out of this trap is through self-compassion, but that this can be challenging if you don't have a strong sense of your own inherent worth. Kristen Neff has done significant research on self-compassion and argues that it is characterized by self-kindness, a sense of common humanity and mindfulness, which, together, "create a self-compassionate frame of mind" (Neff, 2003, p. 212). She highlights that self-compassion is strongly connected to psychological, emotional, physical, and spiritual wellbeing. From an educator perspective, we know that self-compassion is linked to the professional maturity associated with mediating positive relationships with others, emotional intelligence, and wisdom (Neff, 2009a; 2009b).

From an individual perspective, Flowers and Stahl (2011) explain the importance of self-compassion, noting, "The identity of unworthiness is formed of self-blame and a deluge of self-judgments offered by an inner critic who wants nothing to do with self-compassion. It's far more interested in masochistic endeavours like self-improvement projects that it's never satisfied with. But this just gets you more stuck in feeling deficient for several reasons, the foremost being the very idea that there's a faulty and unworthy self that needs improvement" (p. 93). How do we avoid this culture of blame and shame that emerges from an over-reliance on critical self-improvement stemming from a sense of unworthiness? Attuning to the stories that we use to narrate our interpretation of our experiences, growing our habit of awareness and learning to use an appreciative and compassionate lens can offer respite. We can do this through practicing mindful awareness with a focus on compassion and remembering that, "living in the present moment doesn't mean that you discard your goals. . . . It means remaining oriented to the here and now as you work toward what you want" (Flowers & Stahl, 2011, p. 93). One way of practicing these habits of attention, awareness and a focus on compassion is through the use of meditation. Research has found that engaging in loving-kindness meditations, where you focus your attention toward love, acceptance, and peace for self, for your relations, and for all others, can change the neural pathways in your brain and grow your ability to enjoy life more fully (Davidson, 2003; Fredrickson, 2009). In the next section, we describe a practice we have used with educators as a writing meditation, focusing our attention on what makes us work well, and feel alive and whole in our work.

MINDFUL ART PRACTICE FOR ATTENDING TO STRENGTHS AND PURPOSE: APPRECIATIVE REFLECTIONS

Through the practice of meditation we can grow our capacities for noticing and appreciating the best of who we are and of those around us. We have used a reflection practice with educators that can be understood as a kind of loving-kindness meditation practice which combines images, words, and feelings that inspire love and kindness. Loving-kindness meditations are important to developing attention to flourishing because the meditation is a reminder that self-love and love for our communities go hand in hand. As we become more self-aware of our self as deserving of loving attention we see the value for others. Noticing the connection between how we treat our self and how we treat others will yield great insights. This is a powerful meditation that can be repeated often and when needed. Education is about caring relationships. Considering these relationships through a practice of mindful reflection can help set the intention to live with more positive emotion.

When I am at My Best: A Meditation

Ask colleagues, in an email or in person, to provide you with stories of when they see you at your best at work. Ask them to describe this in as much detail as they can. You can offer to reciprocate. We think you'll find this exercise to be immediately rewarding (in your personal life too) as you read back the positive stories provided to you, and share with others the ways you see them living out their best selves at work.

We have tried this exercise with students in a teacher education program and they reported back that it was a wonderful exercise for seeing themselves in a positive way through the eyes of their family, friends, and colleagues. Carrying out personal assessments and reflections of when you are flourishing are important aspects of gaining greater awareness of who you are and what you value and hold to be important in your work so that you can start to work from these places of strength and value. As you do, you might find that you are able to make sense of your work from a place of meaning, noticing how you use your language and your thoughts to create a narrative about your work that reflects a commitment to values and purpose.

A Letter to My Future Self: A Meditation

The mindful reflection activity of writing a letter to "the future you" was designed to create an opportunity for systems-thinking, an approach for seeing the interconnectedness of the parts that create the whole. Writing a letter to the future was a strategy we used to create an awareness of different perspectives from within the school district system as principals, superintendents, teachers were given the opportunity to read and reflect on each other's visions.

Task: "Imagine you have the power to shape the future. Paint a picture of future that captures the energy, passion, engagement and hopefulness you desire." The following are several "letters to future educators," written by our research participants.

> *Dear Future Educator,*
> *Here's what I hope for you!*
> *I hope you find balance between your professional life and your personal life. And a balance that works for you (not so-so).*
> *I hope you land in a place that's supportive, where people lift you up when you need it and let you fly when you can.*
> *I hope you focus on what you are good at. We often want to be good at everything but pick one or two things and master them. Only then can you take on new things.*
> *I hope you don't worry too much about things that are beyond your control. I want you to believe that you can change the world, but change it in your way. There are parts of the world that we can't change and we shouldn't just focus on that.*
> *I hope you find your people. Even if they are different from you and drive you nuts. You will know that they are your people. And don't worry if you lose them for a bit, you will find your people again.*

> *Dear Future Educator, this is what we dream for you . . .*

- *you are valued.*
- *your unique skills are embraced and celebrated.*
- *you value your students and their unique skills are embraced and celebrated.*
- *your environment is welcoming.*
- *your schedule is flexible and open and shifting so you can grab opportunities for learning in new ways.*
- *content takes a back seat/truck box/trailer distant priority to skills and competencies.*
- *your students are curious and eager to explore and learn.*
- *you are relaxed and happy to be at work.*
- *you have a home life.*
- *you do not have work stresses that invade your home life.*
- *you flourish, you belong, you bloom, you go to seed (in the best way!) and new blooms explore around you.*

In the future ideal flourishing school you will need to pay attention to the following things . . .

Ways of thinking

- *Growth mindset*
- *Willing to take risks*
- *Embrace constraints as opportunities*
- *Relentless in thought, and toward achieving goals (persistence, resilience)*
- *Playful and curious*

Colleague relations

- *Colleague co-plan/co-learn and play together*
- *Hierarchy is flattened*
- *Opportunities for relationship-building*
- *Trust and protection from judgment*
- *Respecting of alternative views and tensions*

Leadership

- *Shared responsibility*
- *Creates a safe space for risk-taking*
- *Foster leadership in others*
- *Constantly looking for skills and talents in others*

- *Engage and connect with all the stakeholders to truly understand needs*

System

- *Reduced confinement of structures (block rotation, room allocation, etc.)*
- *Opportunity for teacher collaboration within the day*
- *Greater connection and access to the larger community (what would happen if you changed school goals to "community goals"?)*

Yours truly, Classroom Teacher 2021

Dear Superintendent of 2021:

Well, it has been quite a journey for everyone in the district. We learned that the foundations of a flourishing school are strength-based (not deficit-based), belonging-based (not isolated), engagement in purposeful work (not just compliance), and experiencing our work lives as a whole (not fragmented).

We began applying these foundations by identifying our strengths which are many. We have support staff and professional staff that are creative, committed, and focused on meeting the needs of the students in our district. We identified that there is a strong desire within these dedicated people to work together to create a new sense of team within each school and the district. We determined that we don't want our work and school lives to be just about compliance and filling in the workday, but that we want our work to be meaningful and produce real results that we can be proud of. We also identified that we want our work to be part of the inclusive whole in the district and not have a sense of being fragmented from this central focus.

We brought representatives together from all of our "partners" (and I am proud to use that word!) to discuss how we could ensure that everything we do is built on these foundations. We established a Partner Advisory Council to formally bring our partners together and defined what collaboration, openness, and transparency really mean and established processes for how this group would work together.

Our leadership team of trustees, central staff, district management, principals, and vice principals share a common vision of strategic priorities and communicate effectively about our progress toward these objectives. We support effective educational programs and ensure that our district is working as efficiently as possible toward these priorities.

This process has not been easy and has required time, honesty, and trust as we have walked down this road. Although this has sometimes led to difficult conversations, I can say that the end result has been that we are a district that reflects our core values in a much more authentic way in how we treat each other day to day. It has required old foundations to be broken, and a spirit of forgiveness instilled recognizing that mistakes will be made as we travel on this road together. We recognize now that trust, hope, and compassion are the virtues that are the core of every thriving organization.

The key for us in going on this journey was to commit to the specific behaviors that were required to move this discussion from theory to practice. Defining our own meaning for the three domains of the framework was our first conversation: leaderful mindsets, adaptive inquiry, and subjective wellbeing are powerful concepts but we had to define them in our own terms to make them accessible to everyone in the organization and in the community. We then listed the specific behaviors that the organization would need to adopt and commit to for each of these domains. We revisit these commitments whenever we get together to remind ourselves of being consistent in their application.

Along the way we have made mistakes to be sure, but we have been able to overcome these with forgiveness and then persistence. Our teachers and support staff are truly thriving as we have established new foundations and created this common culture in our schools. The possibilities for continued growth into new areas are limitless as we learn more and adopt new behaviors consistent with the flourishing framework.

Our future is bright indeed as we flourish together and thrive together.

What these educators shared is that to feel a sense of flourishing, they and their students, need to feel, connect, share, and learn how to be well together. These letters are examples of the stories that emerged from these educators as they were invited to reflect from an appreciative and open mind and heart, where they focused on what matters most to them in their work, what makes them come alive and thrive. From their stories we learned that flourishing is relational, connected to the educators' personal strengths, to their higher purposes, and to their focus on practices that fostered and supported their wellbeing. In the next chapter, we share an example of an organizational strategy, job crafting, that can be useful for intentionally designing your work, where you can, in ways that contribute to more fully enjoying life at work and in in ways that promote meaningful opportunities for connection and learning for you and your students.

Chapter Five

Job Crafting

Throughout this book we have offered that an educator's mindful alignment develops through ongoing, mindful, professional learning. Specifically, growing mindful awareness of wellbeing, positive relationships, and strengths, passions, and purposes through practicing the arts provided—and many others that we know educators already practice—can nurture mindful alignment as we learn to craft a self, over and over again, that reflects our best intentions. We suggest that practicing mindful arts for growing aware- ness as a professional learning endeavor can support a person's capacity to influence the development of their work systems in ways that foster greater wellbeing. Our work with educators reveals that those who become more mindfully aware find themselves more capable of influencing organizational adaptations that then better harness the strength of people within the organ- ization.

In this chapter, *job crafting* is described as an organizational strategy that provides educators with opportunities to set themselves up for meaningful accomplishments in the system within which they work. Job crafting is the act of designing the work of teaching from and with the educator's perspec- tive. It is a term that refers to an individual's tendency and tenacity, within the boundaries of their job, to arrange work activities, routines, and attitudes about work to elicit a sense of meaning, purpose, passion, and personal satisfaction from their work (Wrzesniewski & Dutton, 2001). When we at- tune through a lens of appreciation to wellbeing, positive perceptions, posi- tive relationships, and our higher purpose, we can notice spaces where we do have autonomy for making meaningful decisions about how to craft our work in ways that empower us to practice the art of living with wellbeing at the center of our work and lives, listening and connecting in positive relation- ships, and living from our strengths. Through this book we have described

67

that there is no one way that fits all processes for developing mindful alignment as a strong foundation for a life of personal and professional flourishing. The same goes for job crafting. There is no right or wrong way to craft one's job; what is important is that job crafting be a responsive and ethical act that meets the needs of the teacher and the community. Job crafting is possible when teachers can attend to relational-living as a way of co-creating their work, and of crafting within community a self that reflects ongoing attention to working and living from a sense of wholeness, from intentions and actions that nurture mind, body, and spirit.

In many schools the administrative leadership team designs teachers' job allocations without detailed consultation with the individual teachers. Sometimes such structures limit teachers' decision making, and can frustrate or block their sense of professional autonomy and discernment. This can then lead to a feeling that work expectations are overly imposed and beyond the teacher's control, and can contribute to a loss of motivation for the teacher. From our research, we know that teachers thrive when they are mindfully aware of self and others, and know where they are able to make differences in the lives of their students and their families through using their strengths. Attending to work from a perspective of job crafting means that teachers can use their knowledge of their strengths and capacities, and organize their jobs with meeting the various and multiple needs of their learning community. This kind of job organization might involve two teachers working together and making the decision to split their tasks in light of each other's strengths. Teachers may create place-based programs specifically to meet the needs of students, and these programs might be facilitated by teachers who self-identify an interest in the program given their passion and strength. Job sharing scales self-awareness and our subjective wellbeing up and out into the learning community and can help build adaptive communities. In adaptive communities, educators work together to build organizational structures, space, and mindsets for providing opportunity for co-created approaches to teaching in ways that make sense to their community (Cherkowski, & Walker, in progress).

MINDFUL ALIGNMENT FROM AN
ORGANIZATIONAL PERSPECTIVE

We see mindful alignment as integral to co-constructing an organization that truly values wellbeing and therefore as a skill that would be compatible with a move toward job crafting in schools. Margaret Wheatley is an organizational scholar who informs our growing awareness of the importance of organizing our schools and other workplaces from an intention of flourishing as an essential guiding principle. She writes, "it is time to become passionate about what's best in us and to create organizations that welcome in our creativity, contribution, and compassion" (Wheatley, 2015, p. 57). As we have described, we see that flourishing at work is something we can actively construct on our own, and even more powerfully with others.

Collective job crafting can improve commitment, job satisfaction, and performance when groups change the way they work to enable increases in engagement in behaviors that align with their preferences, passions, strengths, and interests (Leana, Appelbaum, & Shevchuk, 2009). For example, we can collaborate with others in ways that play into each of our strengths. We can develop a habit of noticing what works in our practice and deliberately planning our days to include at least one of these aspects every day in our responsibilities, or making a point of seeking out a little fun and levity with colleagues during breaks in our teaching. There is more to learn about the benefits of job crafting in schools. At this point, we do see that job crafting is a possible outcome of mindful alignment, to develop habits of mind that contribute to a more generative set of stories about our work that inform and lead us toward noticing how we live out our higher purpose in our work.

MINDFUL ALIGNMENT: A TOOL FOR CRAFTING OUR SELVES AND OUR WORK COMMUNITIES

We are currently living in a time of rapid change and of significant upheaval and turmoil across the globe as communities and societies react and respond to economic, environmental, and cultural challenges. We experience the frustration, anxiety, and even trauma that comes with living in these uncertain times, and we are in need of new ways of coping with the massive challenges facing humanity. To cope with the increasing rates and complexity of change, with the increasingly diverse and globalized communities within which we live and work, and to meet the growing economic, cultural environmental, and political challenges facing the future, we need new tools to aid us in finding new solutions and new ways forward. Many in the leadership and organization world have been writing about these needs for adaptive leadership that will help guide us through collective problem-solving in a more flexible, open minded, and collaborative way. We have seen that mindful alignment is a model of self, team, and organizational learning that takes this notion of responsive learning one step further. Otto Scharmer (2009) suggests that the strongest organizational learning tends to be a reframing of the learning garnered from experience to provide novel solutions to complex challenges. However, he notes that there is a level of learning that is possible, but rarely accessed, that would provide learning insights into the future as it is emerging, and that these insights contain the wisdom for knowing and doing required for the increasingly complex challenges facing our world. He provides a model of learning that recognizes the potential of accessing a broad sense of awareness and presence that is available in each individual and in each system. What is often missing is a deeper level of awareness. Individuals and collectives rarely access the field of awareness from which action originates, and so we are hindered in our change plans and strategies by our *blind spot*, our inability to access a deeper level of learning. Within this field of awareness, limitless creativity is possible, and so is the potential for developing together new ways forward in these increasingly uncertain time. Scharmer (2009) explains his view that we are at a crossroads of learning; we can do as we have always done, or we can pay attention to the new possibilities that he sees are available if we pay attention:

> What, then, is arising from the rubble? How can we cope with these shifts? What I see rising is a new form of presence and power that starts to grow spontaneously from and through small groups and networks of people. It's a different quality of connection, a different way of being present with one another and with what wants to emerge. When groups begin to operate from a real future possibility, they start to tap into a different social field from the one they normally experience. It manifests through a shift in the quality of thinking, conversation, and collective action. When that shift happens, people can connect with a deeper source of creativity and knowing and move beyond the patterns of the past. They step into their real power, the power of the authentic self. I call this change a shift in the social field because that term designates the totality and type of connections through which the participants of a given system relate, converse, think and act. (p. 4)

Acknowledging the importance of individuals and groups in engaging from an authentic self and thinking about change as a process of collectively tapping into a social reality from which the future may emerge is a new way to think about change in schools and organizations. We have shared through this book our beliefs about the importance of placing the cultivation of the authentic self at the heart of the work of teaching, learning, leading in schools, and provided theory and practices for attuning to how we are expressing our authentic self at work and in life through the practices designed to cultivate mindful alignment, the foundation for human flourishing.

JOB CRAFTING:
A TRANSFORMATIVE SOCIAL LEARNING PROCESS

The challenges of our time are calling to us to move in new ways so that we can rise up to the best of who we hope to be individually and collectively. Scharmer (2009) describes that "we haven't been able to create schools and institutions of higher education that develop people's innate capacity to sense and shape their future, which I view as the single most important capability for this century's knowledge and co-creation economy" (p. 3). He argues for new social processes of learning to harness potential for transformation that is currently dormant in most individuals and organizations, our consciousness, the deep space within each of us from which comes our best possibilities and creativity (p. 95). We suggest that as teachers develop their mindful alignment, they can tap into this consciousness and begin crafting their professional life in new and generative ways.

We have described that within schools there is sometimes the assumption that a teacher's work happens through the vision and goals of a formal leader who then influences others to work with them to carry out the necessary actions to reach the desired goal. In contrast, Scharmer (2009) suggests (and we agree) that leaders can be considered as "all people who engage in creating change or shaping their future, regardless of their formal positions in institutional structures" (p. 5) and that what counts most in terms of the work of leadership is "not only what leaders do and how they do it but their 'inner condition.' The inner place from which they operate or the source from which all of their actions originate" (p. 7). We think that practicing mindful alignment can help educators to notice the stories that shape who they have been, and attend more deeply to the stories that can frame who they hope to become in ways that empower them to move forward authentically and with a sense of purpose and meaning. This is a holistic, fluid, and evolving process and not a step-wise approach to change; however, we would like to offer an example from the experience of our research team member who will show how her attention to mindful alignment worked to recraft and reshape her role as a classroom teacher in order to utilize the skills she was developing and deeming essential to wellbeing in schools. As a way of providing a practical example of how mindful alignment can serve as a model of shifting how we organize and carry out our work as educators, we offer an example from Kelly's reflective research notes as a teacher when she was undertaking an inquiry with her teaching partner to craft their work in a different way, to highlight and foreground the importance of inquiry-based teaching using mindfulness as a primary strategy for growing relationships and meaningful awareness in the classroom. This example provides a brief glimpse into how it might look for educators to job craft in their own work from an intention of growing flourishing for self, students, and all others in their learning community. Through this example, we highlight how attending to the three aspects of mindful alignment—wellbeing, relationships, strengths, and purpose—can open mind, body, and spirit for transforming teaching and learning for flourishing.

JOB CRAFTING: AN EDUCATOR'S EXPERIENCE

In 2016/2017, my teaching partner and I decided to organize our teaching job in a way that we felt enabled us to create an inquiry-based classroom. This was not our first collaboration. In fact leading up to the school year, we had the opportunity to develop a mindful teaching and philosophy together (Hanson, 2017). This mindful practice included sitting together for breath meditation practices and contemplative conversations through which we shared what we noticed as we developed awareness of our wellbeing, our relationships, and our strengths (qualities of mindful alignment). Through this collaborative process, we came to a place of greater self-awareness, and we believed we could create a learning environment that was designed to honor the integrity of our inquiry into mindfulness, and to offer such alignment to our students. With support from our administrators, we created the following commitments as the beginnings of our planning:

- To learn, we emphasize self-understanding and personal growth.
- We acknowledge that all members of the classroom have multiple identities.
- We recognize that all members need care.
- We learn through inquiry.
- We share our learning with our community.
- We learn from our community.
- We learn through various ways of knowing.

These actionable intentions were the foundation of our co-planning, co-teaching, and assessment, and they emerged from our renewed sense of self/other/strengths. From these commitments we began what became our first efforts at job crafting. The first thing we designed was a flexible timetable. We let go of having a timetable with times set to teach specific subjects in favor of an integrated day. The only pieces of the whole school schedule that we followed were the times for lunch and recess. We knew that we wanted a more integrated approach to our day because of our holistic understanding of wellbeing, and so we made an intention to take an integrated approach to our teaching for this desire of wholeness, of wellbeing.

Holistic Wellbeing as a Teaching Intention

We wanted students to learn holistically through a sense of how all aspects of learning are connected. Our educational aim was the ongoing nurturing of competent, caring, loving, and lovable people, and we felt that many of the barriers from the system that we had previously felt in our teaching could be understood as false, as barriers that we identified and maintained through our beliefs about what it means to be a teacher in a system. We had felt that much of the frustration that we had felt around what we perceived as barriers in learning that enforced binary and limited views of knowledge and the world could be shifted if we shifted our mindsets and as many of the organizational structures as we could. The first start was shifting the timetable for our students to reflect an integrated, holistic approach to teaching and learning where we would engage in inquiry-based learning projects that cut across many aspects of the curriculum and that could be followed in a deeper way with a timetable that honored their learning, as opposed to the truncated timetable we had been experiencing that honored the binding of classroom learning according to subject areas.

We also wanted students to focus more on their current experiences, to be more present in the learning, rather than going along with preestablished beliefs about subject matter and themselves as learners. We wanted the students to inquire into who they are as learners as to make sense of learning as active knowledge constructors, not as passive recipients of prescribed sets of facts and activities. We believe that education should provide a grounding for people to recognize their potential, and to learn how to support and contribute to growing the potential in others, believing that when we grow and change as individuals we grow and change as a community. We believe that as a species, to transform from surviving to thriving, we must discover and uncover who we are with both curiosity and compassion, and that these insights need a platform to be created in community, and also to be shared with others. With these aims in mind, we dedicated ourselves to developing our classroom as an open and negotiable forum to investigate our potential, our values, and to learn to value and engage with the experiences of others. In offering our classroom in this way, we as learners (teachers and students), engaged in fostering a community for continuous exploration.

The start of opening myself to these new approaches to teaching, such as an integrated timetable, was learning to notice myself holistically. For example, I noticed that I was experiencing feelings of being overwhelmed by my own expectations of myself as a science, math, English, etc., teacher. I had concerns of exhaustion, of feeling overwhelmed, and of not honoring my intentions to teach people, not subjects. However, despite these concerns, I was agreeing to take on more and more within these separate domains, even though what I was agreeing to were not tasks that I felt best nurtured my students' needs.

For me, noticing moments when I am *in contradiction* is a particularly powerful alignment process. Through mindful alignment my teaching becomes a consciousness-elevating practice. In order to craft a teaching job in ways that honor my teaching values requires a deep level of self-community awareness, so that decisions can be made that meet the needs of the community. It is also important to note that not all contradictions need to be worked through. As I am more self-reflective in my work I notice my own limitations and am aware of these blindspots. While I may not be able to work out the contradiction, this awareness helped me to be more open and flexible with my perspective because I realized that there is much that I cannot see or understand at any given moment. I was able to offer myself compassion in those moments of contradiction because I could see with greater awareness of various influences of the system, that it was not a personal failure but was an aspect of the organization. This awareness offered new perspectives on my work that allowed me to pause, reflect, and frame a story about my work in ways that helped me to move forward in an appreciative, generative, and soul-keeping way. I believe that all genuine learning requires an open approach, a willingness to engage in invention and reinvention, and I wanted to craft my work in ways that honored this space. Through mindful alignment I was not simply reinventing my experience to serve what I believed, but it helped me leave space for what is still unknown and to build collaborative relationships to test and share my ideas.

Relationships

Honoring relationships is another quality of mindful alignment that we describe in this book. Listening to the relationships around me was another process that supported my move toward job crafting. If I wanted to reinvent my job to be more responsive to the community, I needed to collaborate deeply, and with people from a variety of perspectives. Attending to relationships through listening allowed me to create more respect and understanding in the groups I work in. It helped me maintain a greater state of presence for creating a dialogical approach to teaching and designing.

I found that as I grew my capacity for listening through mindfulness practices when I communicated with people without being reactive or without judgment I could cultivate a deeper level of social presence. Scharmer (2009) wrote about presencing, suggesting that this state can occur in situations where people interact from a place of self-clarity, which comes from being connected to your ideals and self. It was from this place of presence and awareness that our teaching commitments became actions. From a state of presence learning from inquiry seems to come more naturally. To promote inquiry learning, I had to become more aware of my values, and my actions. For example, I realized that I did not need to be in control of the learning, and that ideas need to be explored and questioned by many in the community. I learned that I could embrace new ideas rather than trying to force my ideas from the past to fit my current learning needs. This gentle positioning of values did not mean that I lost my conviction. Rather, I found confidence to move forward in my values. I found when I developed deep listening, that communication became stronger and deeper bonds were created with my students and with my colleagues. When you are deeply listening to people, they feel safe and valued. In dialogue and in the social field of presence, challenging conversations are welcomed and necessary to propel transformative learning. In my work, I found that if I remained committed to not judging, that the conversations deepened and that a more transformative learning experience was possible for me, and for those with whom I was in relationship.

The following reflective letter sums up our experiences during our year of job crafting. This reflection speaks to the strengths we brought forward in ourselves and our students throughout the year.

Dear Parents,

What made this year of teaching so rewarding? While there were many factors, they all relate to the joy of witnessing learning. Student learning looked like students asking questions and being excited to be at school. One way we knew our students were excited to learn was when they took ownership of planning activities for the class. Each morning the students (different ones, at different times) met in the classroom before school and discussed the day ahead, and part of this ritual was writing the agenda for the day and inspirational quotes on the board. So many days started with a pre-lesson because there were so many questions and insights that arose just from discussing the plans for the day. So many mornings we would hear, *This is going to be a great day.* Or, *I am really looking forward to this.*

This year taught us that student learning looks like students' voice. We knew the students were learning and growing as their own individual being-ness came into focus. The students expressed who they are, what their preferences are, what they struggle with, how they deal with those struggles. We saw our role as to help students stretch and reflect on their claims.

The voices grew as the students grew in confidence over the year and we believe this growth was because our classroom learning was grounded in a climate of nurturing gratitude, community, and strengths. Our students were learning as the result of the complicated ways the students were weaving their sense of gratitude and freedom and collaboration into their storytelling and their play and their inquiry.

The stories the students wrote and told were an explosion of dialogue, and art, and doodles and the characters came alive through animation and puppetry. This year we read a lot, and the teachings from our readings also led our charge; we marched as we carried buckets of water from the creek, imagined different lives at the global schoolhouse, scoured the museum for treasures, and ate the foods from many different cultures. We had unstructured play time every afternoon. During this time, the students all played together. This play ebbed and flowed from tag games, to swing games, to ping pong, and four square. In these games the students always added their rules and flare.

Some of the greatest play of all happened in science. In science, the possibility of creation unleashed the deepest sense of wonder and adventure. We had to start again so many times—for example, the bumper car ramp was not steep enough or fast enough, and the poly balls did not bounce. In each case, we (teachers) stepped aside as in-depth discussions around the table erupted and students met to re-read, re-do, make better, and problem solve together. The stories and play and the layers of inquiry were truly never ending.

Throughout the last term, we wrote parallel universe stories. These stories reminded us that things are not always as they seem and that things can always be different. On our rained-out payday, we watched the movie *The Neverending Story*, an awesome example of a parallel universe story. *The Neverending Story* depicts the fight against the nothingness which is the emptying of the imagination. The movie depicts the fight for the survival of all the alternate worlds created from reading books in the minds and hearts of the reader. These worlds of imagination were alive and well in our classroom.

Alongside our fantastic imaginings, we understood that it matters how we story our lives, that language matters, that what we do matters. We knew the power of the language of appreciation, and that was so crucial to our learning and growing. Through appreciation we acknowledged and valued each other, expressed our ideas, and gave feedback. Through the language of appreciation, we described things in new ways and we can problem solve.

Seeing so much student learning made this a rewarding year of teaching. The level of engagement that we are describing that fills the heart, truly rested on the professional development that was happening alongside the unfolding of the learning in the classroom. We engaged rigorously in our learning about the nature and calling of teaching over the course of the year, and we are so grateful for the opportunity to work together this year.

Finally, we know that deep student learning and engagement is fueled at home and through family support and we are so grateful for your involvement and feedback and partnerships.

Thank you so much for a wonderful year, and we wish you much wellness along the never-ending story of learning.

Sincerely,
Your teachers

Through my job crafting experience, I learned that a sense of wellbeing increases as students, teachers, and other school leaders continue to learn and challenge themselves to grow more of what they know makes them well. Mindful alignment nurtured my learning and my self-confidence.

Learning to Notice and Work from Our Strengths

My teaching partner and I crafted our job into the integrated, emergent model we have described in some detail here because we believe in our own strengths of observation and dedication to our values. When our job became the living actions of those strengths, our love of our job escalated and so did our sense of flourishing. As others seek to improve their wellbeing and the wellbeing of others in their work environment by attuning to positive perceptions, positive relationships, and focusing on higher purpose, we hope that they may also find their work environment becoming more engaging. In the workplace, Ben-Shahar (2009) maintained that "happiness and success do go together" (p. 148). Models, or examples, such as this one, of educators living out mindful alignment toward the aim of flourishing can empower others to also attune to the stories that shape and construct their realities and that influence how they cultivate positive relationships and live from their strengths and a higher purpose.

MINDFUL ALIGNMENT: BEYOND JOB CRAFTING

As we have shared throughout this book, we are influenced by writing and research that encourages us to notice and nurture the beauty, strength, and virtue in each of us as the professional learning journey that is at the heart of what it means to be a teacher. Job crafting is one possible outcome of mindful alignment, but as we have been learning about the impact of positive and appreciative states of mind in how we engage in our work and life, we believe that others who take up the challenge and call to flourish will come to find other creative and life enhancing outcomes. As we worked with our participants to understand from them what it means to flourish in their work, we heard the message loud and clear that educators are pressed for time and energy, that there is already so much to do in their work, that they don't have time to add on more of anything, even if that work may lead them to flourish. We recognized that teachers have been conditioned over the years to assume that they should look outside to find the answers to how to improve their practice, that these answers will be given to them after they take a workshop or attend an in-service program intended to professionally develop their deficiencies. Research on school improvement is catching up and catching on to this sense of frustration from educators that working to fix them and their practice by sending them to or bringing in an outsider expert is not effective (Cochran-Smith & Lytle, 1993; 2009; Hoban, 2010). Finding ways for educators to develop mindful alignment with their colleagues is an important shift in school improvement, and we eagerly support further research on how to encourage and engage teachers in these efforts.

Within this mindful alignment model, we want to suggest a shift in the lens that we use to view our practice, toward an appreciative and positive one. As we have been sharing, mindful alignment encourages a focus on an appreciative lens regarding school improvement—looking for ways that we already engage in work routines and habits that support our flourishing, and then finding ways to get more of this in our work. This is not an add-on or additional skill to learn, and is not about repairing deficiencies or mending broken practices or spirits. Rather, this inquiry is a life-long learning journey undertaken with colleagues, toward supporting the best and highest in ourselves and in others at work. This professional learning journey can be carried out as a process of deepening self-awareness to attend and attune to the alignment of our values and intentions for who we hope to become with thoughts, actions, and stories of our experiences. We provided examples in this book of arts, or approaches, for change that empower and enable us to focus our gaze inward to notice what works well, what makes us come to life in our work, and then to mindfully shift our attention toward these existing practices, so that we can emphasize and amplify these flourishing practice and moments in our work.

With our research participants, we noticed that as we engaged with them to learn about the practices that help them to come alive in their work they could look at their teaching in a new way, searching for the best of what already happens. As they carried out this appreciative archaeology of their work, they noticed that they felt energized and excited about much of what was going on at work for them. They appreciated moments of connection with colleagues, moments of laughter and fun in the staff room, times of deep engagement with their students, and times of connecting personally and meaningfully with students and their parents. One of the teachers was quite animated as he shared how, as he was asked to think about practices at work that bring out the best of who he is and help him to feel a sense of engagement and connection at work. He said, "I find inspiration all over. Overall, in different areas, such as inspiration from a colleague or from a program that inspires me to do things differently and from the children and their excitement for learning. It might inspire me to do something new or try a different idea that I didn't even think of, but they inspired me to do something. Everywhere." As the participants talked with each other about their work, they noticed that they appreciated the simple act of taking time to reflect on their work from a positive perspective, in the company of their colleagues. Taking time to be present with our teaching practice by ourselves is important, doing this with our colleagues can be transformative.

We have enjoyed and valued the opportunity to serve as "story catchers" (Baldwin, 2005) for our research participants, learning from them about descriptions and examples of flourishing. As we worked with educators in schools, we noticed the power of positive narrative for transforming themselves and their school organizations as they inquired into what it means to flourish in their work. From our research, we have learned about what it means to organize schools in ways that support flourishing, and continue to grow our understanding about the importance of wellbeing (personal and collective), mindsets for leading for flourishing and creating adaptive communities built on care, trust, and belonging as essential organizational domains for creating spaces and places where educators and their students thrive.

As we continue to build our research story of what it means to flourish in school organizations, we invite you to join with others in a larger conversation toward building theory and practice for positive education. Students, parents, and staff members are part of a growing movement to develop and support flourishing across many school contexts. We encourage those in school learning communities to share their stories with others and to collectively dream their way forward into becoming the best imaginable. We encourage you to work with your colleagues in carrying out flourishing inquiries for the work of school improvement, and to engage with students, parents, and community members in this inquiry, sharing what is learned with others in the larger educational community. In our last chapter, we return to flourishing and the importance of building mindful alignment as foundational for flourishing in schools.

Chapter Six

Mindful Awareness
as a Foundation for Flourishing

We hold the view that humans have a level of agency for constructing, or crafting, their social world. From this social constructionist perspective, we see that the world that we live in is a storied world, with multiple scripts that shape the way we live and experience our lives. Through practicing the arts of mindful alignment we can learn to notice and inquire into the stories that shape us, those we create, and those that are perhaps pre-scripted for us, passed down and passed along from others. As we grow our capacity for this mindful awareness and alignment of our beliefs and values with our actions and responses, we will move closer toward living an expression of our truest, authentic self. Paying attention to our wellbeing, to the ways we engage in relationships, to how we are expressing our unique passions and strengths, and noticing how our beliefs align with our lived experiences is an ongoing learning process. Over time, this mindful inquiry into who we are and who we hope to become can contribute to a sense of wellbeing and of flourishing.

Part of what we are exploring through our theories of and practices for mindful alignment is that every human is born into a storied world, a world filled with cultural traditions, ideas about morality, and assumptions about identity. These inherited stories guide the way we experience education, both as educators and students. The stories contain instructions for organizing the context and content of our school life-worlds. The context, including the physical organization of the school, the timetable, the weekly and monthly calendars, are defined by and contained in these stories. The content of what is learned, what ways there are to share knowledge, what knowledge is deemed important and worthwhile are also reproduced through stories. As humans, from our earliest age, the storied rhythms of educational life shape and position us with a great sense of what ought to be done, said, felt, and believed.

Living in pre-storied, or already storied, ways in schools can be comfortable as we seamlessly move in natural, knowable, patterned, and predictable ways through the life of school, because there can be reassurance and certainty in traditions and well-worn pathways. However, this pre-storied experience can also be disturbing, particularly when the story-world does not acknowledge, or recognize the values and ideas from our various home-settings or from the inner landscapes of our experiences. Educators feel the tension and weight of a pre-storied world that has determined what it means to "do school" each time they are confronted by the need, desire, and voice of their inner person who may not exactly fit the conventional or traditional story. Difference interrupts our certainty, and as educators we may find ourselves in dilemmas where we are disrupted by the disconnections that occur between our lived experiences and our particularly formed expectations. When these gaps are too great, as educators, we may experience a sense of alienation (Macdonald & Shirley, 2009), and a feeling we cannot perform the scripted role of being an educator within the dominant set of conflicting stories. At these times, educators suffer cognitive dissonance and moral injury (Levinson, 2015) from having to choose between supporting the personal needs and the wellbeing of a student or oneself, or of perhaps having to maintain the order, rules, expectations that have been pre-established by the collective, dominant story. While these stories can seem hardwired into the fabric of a school or society and may seem daunting to address, there are always small gaps (Scharmer, 2009) that, once noticed, provide opportunities to uncover a different way of storying our social world.

We have argued that we have influence, or agency, to notice and shift the stories that shape the experiences that make up the life-worlds within which we work and live. Maxine Greene (1978) describes how educators ought to become more wide awake to the landscapes of learning that make up the school life and to our agency within those landscapes. The landscape of learning is diverse, with many realities existing within a classroom and a school culture. Each person brings to the landscape of learning their conceptions and stories based on their own experiences and the relationships that make up who they are. These stories can bump into and contradict other constructions other within the life-world of a school. A dominant Western depiction of learning has been storied as a product of intertwining logic and self-understanding in a world where it is claimed that self can be rationally, logically known. This interpretation of learning and knowing has often dismissed other ways of knowing, including those based in relational, place-based, aesthetic, or other ways of knowing and doing. For educational theorists, like Greene, human beings will live more freely and more joyously when they grapple with the complexity of what it means to know something, to do something, or to be something. She argues that we need to become wide awake to the possibility that traditions of the mind and the stories that promise a reasonable, logical, and orderly world lack the imagination and liminal structures for holding multiple perspectives about what it means to live a human life. These dominant narratives can constrain us and are often insufficient to support a more fulsome development of human experience throughout our lives (Nussbaum, 2011). We see the potential, promise, and benefits in reclaiming a more full human development approach in education, through noticing and attending to how we story teaching, learning, leading, and living well together in schools through mindful alignment practices for attuning to wellbeing, relationships, passions, and strengths.

The work of attuning with mindfulness, to our wellbeing, to how we build relationships, and to living from our passions and strengths as a process for crafting a self that reflects who we are and who we hope to become, can be developed over time and with practice, patience, and love. As we build these practices, we can craft ourselves more and more through an authentic discernment that notices how our values, our intentions, and our desires for who we hope to become are more and more aligned with the actions we perform on our own and with others as we work, live, and learn together. In this way, we are building mindful alignment, a way of being that reflects our attunement to the highest purposes we can imagine for ourselves, aligned with behaviors, responses, and actions.

We understand our social reality as a set of constructions, expressed through language, that reflect a myriad of possible interpretations rather than simply one absolute truth about that experience. From this perspective, we notice how mindfulness can be seen of as a way of learning that leads to a more open, curious, and present sense of experience through "the continuous creation of new categories, openness to new information; and an implicit awareness of more than one perspective" (Langer, 1997, p. 4). Doing this work of crafting the self involves getting curious about the self, noticing and paying attention within the present moment to the inner terrain, the hidden soul. With practice, this curiosity can morph into a habit of deeper awareness as we focus on the three aspects of mindful alignment and notice the alignment of our actions, responses, and behaviors with our beliefs, values, and goals.

This mindful inquiry process is a job that is about the self, but it is not solitary work. We find that, as we do this work, we are better able to connect with others, to build and enjoy the kind of relationships that are vital to our thriving. We also find that as we invite others to join us in this process of better understandings of ourselves, we learn that it is through learning about and understanding the other that we can find opportunities to revisit the self. We notice that a process of mindful inquiry, of noticing, paying attention to and reflecting on the architecture of our hidden soul, is foundational for flourishing for self and others.

MINDFULNESS AS FOUNDATIONAL FOR FLOURISHING IN SCHOOLS

As we have described in our previous writing (Cherkowski & Walker, 2014; 2016), there are many possible descriptions of what it means to flourish and what the antecedents or preconditions for flourishing look like. From a psychological perspective, to *flourish* means "to live within an optimal range of human functioning, one that connotes goodness, generativity, growth, and resilience" (Fredrickson & Losada, 2005, p. 678). Persons who flourish grow in terms of resiliency, self-fulfillment, contentment, and happiness (Haybron, 2008; Martin & Marsh, 2006; Rassmussen, 1999). Conceptions of human flourishing are steeped in ancient moral and ethical roots, from the Aristotelian concept of *eudaimonia*, and understood as the desired and dignified good life for which we all ought to strive (Nussbaum, 1996). Attending to strengths and positive outlooks, as opposed to a deficit-model of thinking, can increase resilience, vitality, and happiness, and can decrease stress, anxiety, and depression (Achor, 2011; Lyubomirsky, 2007; Fredrickson, 2008; Seligman, 2009). From the research, we know that wellbeing at work is closely tied to job satisfaction, to fewer sick days and absences, and to employees putting more thought into their work and being more productive, as well as feeling more fulfilled through their work. Seligman (2011) describes flourishing as the confluence or coming together of positive emotion, engagement, relationship, meaning, and achievement. The National Economics Foundation, a thinktank out of Britain that promotes social, economic, and environmental justice, established five practices of wellbeing: connect, be active, keep learning, take notice, and give.

These definitions and descriptions are helpful, however, we think it is important to understand the ideas of wellbeing in the context of schools. And so, through our research, we aimed to understand what it means to teachers to flourish in their own way so that they could learn to recognize moments of flourishing and build more of them. We gathered stories about the ways educators come to understand and describe the inner workings of their identity. Our research has led us to many engaging and heartfelt conversations with friends, family, and colleagues about various aspects of flourishing. We have encountered many questions within these conversations. Often questions focus on the "how" of flourishing, such as, "How can people bring more flourishing into their lives?" or, "How can we flourish when it seems like so much of our work and life is chaotic, frantic or overwhelming?" Sometimes we are asked "why" questions, such as "Why is it important to understand human flourishing as a way to improve schools?" And sometimes the questions focused on "who." We have noticed that these kinds of questions seem to frame or position flourishing as something outside of the fundamental human condition, as exceptional. Some of these questions sound like: Can just *anybody* describe themselves as flourishing? Who *really* flourishes? How can we *measure* or *judge* who is or is not *really* flourishing? Is flourishing a fiction, a fad, a trait, a state, or perhaps an elusive destination? At the root of these questions seems to be the assumption that aspiring to flourish in our work and life is reserved for certain people, not necessarily for all of us, and that flourishing is somehow out of reach or perhaps not even within our beliefs about what we ought to dream about in our own work and life. We value these questions. In our own ways we have each wrestled with uncertainty in our own work and lives. In part, we wanted to write this book to address the core assumptions underneath these questions: Who ought to strive to flourish, and what does it means to flourish in work and life? Also, what does it mean to foster flourishing in others? We want to offer a new story, one that foregrounds the dignity of striving to understand and infuse a sense of flourishing as integral to cultivating a sense of wholeness, of abundance in everyone's work and in each person's life journey. We see that this shift toward aspiring to thrive, rather than just survive, to be at the heart of our work as educators. We want to assure our readers that flourishing is accessible to us all. We will experience flourishing in our own unique ways and we can support each other to grow in our personal understandings of what it means to flourish and foster flourishing in others.

ENCOURAGING WHOLENESS THROUGH DEVELOPING THE INNER TERRAIN

As described above, our positive lens for research on school improvement has focused on understanding how to cultivate conditions where all members of a community flourish at work, and this has led us to examine and explore the various forces, factors, and conditions that influence and inform what it can mean to flourish in schools (cf. Cherkowski & Walker, 2016; 2014; 2013a; 2013b). Not unexpectedly, we have found that there are many different ways to describe what it means to flourish in our work as educators, and that as we attend to the personal nature of what it means to thrive, we can create more of what it is that makes us feel most alive, engaged, and connected in our work. From educator reports, we hear that flourishing means an aliveness, a sense of connection to the people with whom you work, and with the students in your care. It has been described as a sense of living out your values, and being part of working toward a higher purpose. Purpose in participant descriptions takes on two meanings. Some conceptions of purposeful experiencing of flourishing illustrate the external joy of achieving an end result, the outcome of an established goal, a legacy, a product. Another conception of purpose arises from the experience of being open to the unknown, present and in the moment, being swept away in a flow of learning. Both ways of experiencing purpose are rich, particularly if the achievements and aspirations of work are set out in a way that aligns professional and personal values. What is common from both conceptions of purpose is that feeling a sense of purpose requires a level of self-awareness. Given that feeling a sense of purpose is fundamental to experiences of flourishing, we suggest that, as educators, we need to learn how to grow more self-awareness toward uncovering and living out our purpose at work, and that we need to feel supported in this growth by our organizations.

Indeed, as we talked with educators about their views about how we might organize schools to nurture and sustain flourishing for all members of the learning community, we heard from them that paying attention to their inner terrain—how they craft their best selves—was an important element of how to transform the outer terrain of the school experience. This correlates with much research and writing on the importance of personal development and growth in leadership for meaningful change in organizations (Scharmer, 2009; Scharmer & Kaufer, 2013; Quinn, 2015). Certainly, writers in education (whether in teacher education, professional learning, or educational leadership) consistently emphasize the necessity of knowing who you are as a way of connecting meaningfully with curriculum and the students. To do so enables us to develop meaningful opportunities for authentic learning (Palmer, 1998; Wheatley, 1999; Greene, 1978; Starratt, 2004).

Developing the inner terrain means coming to understand the wholeness and fullness of who we are, what we value, and what we hope to be and do as persons and as educators. This is the work of crafting the self and growing our sense of wholeness in and through our professional lives. This work is foundational to cultivating flourishing lifestyles and flourishing school cultures. While the work of crafting the self seems rather simple, like much of what we have introduced so far, we have come to understand that a sustained, inner learning journey can be a difficult, and sometimes stressful, lifelong endeavor. The inner terrain is not always visible and may be hidden in years and years of storied experiences. Through our work with educators, we have come to admire those who engage in honest and open learning about who they are and who they hope to become. We have seen that as we come to notice, understand, and inquire into the stories that shape who we are and how we work and live, we can script stories that encourage and nurture a sense of flourishing. This ongoing mindful learning journey helps us to uncover the hidden architecture of the soul in education.

PAYING ATTENTION THROUGH THE THREE ASPECTS OF MINDFUL ALIGNMENT

As we already described, building and sustaining positive relationships is key to cultivating and sustaining wellbeing (Fredrickson, 2008; Lyubomirsky, 2007; Seligman, 2011). In our research we have heard similar descriptions from educators who described positive relationships at work as a central feature of what it means to flourish. There is a positive correlation between being involved in a social network—friendships, family, and community—and one's sense of wellbeing and happiness. Whether cultivating new friendships or deepening those we currently have, the improvement of relationships often comes with an improvement in our lives. Graham (2009) writes that "there are positive links between wellbeing and friendships, narrowly defined, and social capital, more broadly defined" (p. 189). As one engages in kind acts, one's mood elevates. A person flourishes if there is someone in their life who accepts them unconditionally. Of course, relationships are fundamental to being human and those with many positive connections have higher wellbeing.

Attending to purpose is also integral to our process of crafting a sense of flourishing through ongoing development of mindful awareness. In Greek, *eudemonia* means finding the "daimon" within. This can mean finding the truest, most perfect form of ourselves, and living in ways that expresses that inner self for the improvement of the community. In other traditions, the ultimate is gained by extinguishing desire, finding unity and communion with nature, the wider universe or a higher spirit, or by satisfying one's ultimate purpose in the universe. From a eudemonic perspective, coming to know and express our highest self in the service of helping others is how we see the work of teaching. This work is about coming to know, understand, and then express the best within each of us for the purpose of facilitating the common, higher, and greatest (*summum bonum*) good that we all seek. Traditionally, there have been ten goods identified with the great good: 1. Pleasing oneself (pleasure); 2. Helping one's self to things (wealth); 3. Sustaining physical fitness (health); 4. Gaining honor, fame, and acceptance in sight of others (honor); 5. Exercising power over others (power); 6. Experiencing peace and contentment (peace); 7. Helping others (love-community); 8. Sustaining the health of one's soul (soul-ish health); 9. Gaining wisdom through the knowledge of truth (wisdom); and 10. Experiencing God or transcendence (Kreeft, 1990, p. 73). As we have learned from educators in our research, we tend to guide students to see the best in themselves and we can even guide them in seeing the best in others so that they might work well together in our classrooms, schools, and beyond. For example, we have heard many stories about teachers knowing the importance of connecting to the

essence of each child as a first and most important step in building relationships for learning with each child. One teacher described,

> Knowing who they are as little people in any grade and making that connec-
> tion with who they are as little people, [knowing] what's going on at home,
> what are they like, and discovering what little quirks about them. I find that the
> other stuff falls into place later after getting to know who they are in just the
> smallest of ways.

What seems more challenging is the idea of working with ourselves, learning
to become aware of and bringing forward the "daimon" within each of us as
educators.

We have found that attending to wellbeing, relationships, passions, and
strengths are important points of focus for attunements to presence and the
cultivation of space, detachment, and openness to multiple perspectives. The
spaciousness of mindfulness is a place of possibility. In light of the pre-
storied nature of human experience, the space and pause of mindfulness is a
way to linger with what is, and move forward in ways that involve an equal
balance of letting go and opening up to new possibilities. The mindful practice of being in the present moment without judgment can allow for a possibility of new-becoming and for noticing old worldviews. There is agency in
this presence that can be denied through merely following the habitual narratives. Mindful awareness to the stories that shape our lives can create more
space for reflection, for connecting, and for thriving. There is a public spiritedness to a mindful journey; mindfulness is a community practice in that the
more deeply we connect to ourselves, the more we are able to connect in an
authentic, respectful, and compassionate way with others. Mindfulness reveals relationships in complex ways; slowing down and paying attention
helps us see all the ways that we share relational connections as part of the
human condition.

This conceptualization of mindful alignment reflects our review of the
research literature on flourishing and mindfulness as well as our work with
educators in schools through our research. Through these professional learning opportunities, and through experiencing our own processes, in and out of
flourishing, we have observed repeated themes and patterns that are reflected
in our model of mindful alignment. For example, the need to return to the
moment, to pay attention to the body, and to learn to honor and value our
truest sense of self are themes in the research literature, with our participants
in our research, and in our own lives as we have aimed to grow our own
experiences of flourishing through mindful awareness. We have learned that
mindfulness can be thought of as a foundational practice for flourishing—an
attuning practice for awareness that leads to a self-awareness of our wholeness; it is a means for bringing ourselves back into congruence and align-

ment. We hope this book has informed, and perhaps even inspired, your learning journey toward mindful alignment. May you be well, may you be healthy, may you be happy, may you be whole.

Appendix:
Developing a Breath Practice

Mindfulness is attention, and it is first and foremost attention to breath. The breath practice has been described as the mindful way. It is the breath that reorients the brain; it is the breath practice that automates the pause. The breath is the human energy and flow and it is through the breath that we cultivate our presence in life. We appreciate this description of cultivating mindfulness through attending to our selves: "By being with yourself . . . by watching yourself in your daily life with alert interest, with the intention to understand rather than judge, in full acceptance of whatever may emerge, because it is there, you encourage the deep to come to surface and enrich your life and consciousness with its captive energies. This is the great work of awareness; it removes obstacles and releases energies by understanding the nature of life and mind. Intelligence is the door to freedom and alert attention is the mother of intelligence" (http://www.maharajnis argadatta.com/).

MINDFUL LISTENING

If you have never tried meditation before, mindful listening is a great place to start. Here are a few things to consider: One of the first aspects of meditation that can bring uncertainty is posture. How should the body be positioned as we meditate? There are many different sources of posture advice for medita-tion. We think that part of the fun of developing a mindful practice is getting to know yourself and following your own uniqueness. This means that it is worthwhile to explore a variety of sources for tips on posture. We offer a few suggestions from our own experiences to get you started.

We suggest you start your meditation practice in a comfortable seated position in a quiet place, although some people prefer to stand or lay down. A comfortable chair where your feet can have both soles connected to the ground can help you feel comfortable and anchored. Rest your shoulders, let them drop, and rest your hands on your thighs. Neck position is very important to maintain a long and healthy practice of meditation. To avoid tension in the neck you can let your spine grow tall and just tilt your chin slightly downward.

The most important awareness in meditation is that there is no right or wrong. Meditation is an opportunity to experience the self without judgment. Thoughts and sensations will come and go throughout your meditation, let them come and go. If your thoughts are distracting you from the breath, try naming what is happening "thinking thoughts" and then return to the breath. You do not have to breathe in any special way. Trust that your body knows what to do. Simply notice.

GUIDED PRACTICE FOR LISTENING

Notice the breath coming in the nostrils and out the nostrils.

After a time of sitting with the breath coming in and out (maybe five full breaths), direct your attention to allowing the sounds around you to come and go.

Let the sounds soothe you, let them swirl around you, let them come and go. When you get distracted, return to those sounds. Let the sounds bring you to the present moment.

Notice each breath coming in and out of the body.

Notice the closest and the farthest sounds.

Notice the breath.

A simple listening meditation is always available to you, for as long or as little a time as you like. Feel free to experience your meditation in a place where the sounds are particularly appealing to you. For example, you might be in a park where birds chirp, in your home, or in your office. Wherever you are, notice and listen to the gentle sounds as you inhale and exhale and know that you are doing so perfectly and wonderfully.

When you are ready, draw your attention back to your surroundings.

GUIDED PRACTICE FOR LOVING-KINDNESS

Loving-kindness meditation uses words, images, and feelings to evoke positive emotion. This is a feeling meditation: feel how loving-kindness feels and notice your feeling as you breath in and out love and goodness.

Imagine that those you include in your meditation will receive the love energy from you and that you will receive this from others. Even in a situation where you feel upset or have difficult feelings, this meditation is a way to refocus on kindness and wellness. Love is always an option.

To begin a loving-kindness meditation, begin by sitting in a comfortable fashion. Begin with visualizing the light that shines from and in your heart, with a kind and tender mind; visualize that your breath in brings more light and love and that this love swells into your heart. As you breath out, you share this love.

Let your mind be open to the colors and imaginings that this visualization may bring.

When you have gotten comfortable with this visualization, imagine yourself. Breathe in and out; you begin with yourself because without loving yourself it is almost impossible to love others. Here is the mantra you can recite for yourself:

> *May I be filled with loving-kindness.*
> *May I be safe from inner and outer dangers.*
> *May I be well in body and mind.*
> *May I be at ease and happy.*

Picture yourself as you are now or as you were as a child. Picture yourself as beloved, as deeply cherished. You may want to design your own mantra for this meditation. Choose words that help you access love, acceptance, and peace. Repeat these phrases, letting the feelings be enjoyed throughout your body and mind.

Practice this meditation until the sense of loving-kindness for yourself grows. Trust the process and try not to judge the time it takes to feel more natural or any contrary feelings that may emerge.

When you feel the cultivated sense of loving-kindness for yourself, draw others into your meditation. Again, using the same mantra as you designed for yourself:

> *May you be filled with loving-kindness.*
> *May you be safe from inner and outer dangers.*
> *May you be well in body and mind.*
> *May you be at ease and happy.*

Let the image and feelings of love and kindness be offered to anyone you choose.

Selected References

Abrams, D. (2016). *Lasting happiness in a changing world: The book of joy*. New York: Viking.

Achor, S. (2011). *The happiness advantage: The seven principles of positive psychology and academic achievement*. Thousand Oaks, CA: Corwin Press.

Baldwin, C. (2005). *Storycatcher: Making sense of our lives through the power and practice of story*. Novato, CA: New World Library.

Ben-Shahar, T. (2009). *The pursuit of perfect: How to stop chasing perfection and start living a richer, happier life*. New York: McGraw-Hill Professional.

———. (2008). *Happier*. New York: McGraw-Hill.

Bentz, V. & Sharpiro, J. (1998). *Mindful inquiry in social research*. Thousand Oaks, CA: Sage Publications.

Bodie, G. D., St. Cyr, K., Pence, M., Rold, M., & Honeycut, J. (2012). Listening competence in initial interactions 1: Distinguishing between what listening is and what listeners do. *International Journal of Listening*, 26, 1–28.

Brown, V. & Olson, K. (2015). *The mindful school leader: Practices to transform your leadership and school*. Thousand Oaks, CA: Sage Company.

Brownell, J. (2013). *Listening: Attitudes, principles, and skills*. New York: Pearson.

Buber, M. (1970). *I and thou*. (W. Kaufmann, Trans.). London, UK: Collins Clear-Type Press. (Original work published 1947).

Campbell, J. (1949). *The hero with a thousand faces*. Novato, CA: New World Library.

Cherkowski, S. & Walker, K. (In press). *Teacher wellbeing: Flourishing in schools by noticing, nurturing and sustaining*. Burlington, ON: Word and Deed Publishing.

———. (2017). Educational research as flourishing: Contributing to a pipeline of wellbeing. Published online in the *Canadian Journal of Teacher Research*, www.teacherresearch.ca.

———. (2016). Flourishing leadership: Engaging purpose, passion, and play in the work of leading schools. *Journal of Educational Administration*, 54, 378–392.

———. (2014). Flourishing communities: Re-storying educational leadership using positive research lens. *International Journal of Leadership in Education: Theory and Practice*, 17, 200–217.

———. (2013a). Schools as sites of human flourishing: Musing on an inquiry into efforts to foster sustainable learning communities. *Journal of Educational Administration and Foundations*, 23, 139–154.

———. (2013b). Living the flourishing question: Positivity as an orientation for the preparation of teacher candidates. *Northwest Journal of Teacher Education*, 11, 801–803.

Cherkowski, S., Hanson, K., & Kelly, J. (2015). Living collaborative leadership: Cultivating a mindful approach. In K. Ragoonaden (Ed.), *Mindful teaching and learning: Developing a pedagogy of wellbeing*, pp. 49–67. Lanham, MD: Lexington Books.

Cherkowski, S., Hanson, K., & Walker, K. (Under review). Flourishing in adaptive community: Balancing structures and flexibilities. *Journal of Professional Capital and Community* (submitted September 22, 2017).

Cherkowski, S. & Schnellert, L. (2017). Exploring teacher leadership in a rural, secondary school: Reciprocal learning teams as a catalyst for emergent leadership. *International Journal of Teacher Leadership*, 8(1), 6–25.

Cochran-Smith, M. & Lytle, S. (1993). *Inside/outside: Teacher research and knowledge*. New York: Teachers College Press.

———. (2009). *Inquiry as stance: Practitioner research for the next generation*. New York: Teachers College Press.

Coghlan, A. T., Preskill, H., & Tzavaras Catsambas, T. (2003). An overview of appreciative inquiry in evaluation. *New Directions for Evaluation*, 100, 5–22.

Cooperrider, D. & Srivastva, S. (1987). Appreciative inquiry in organizational life. *Research in Organizational Change and Development*, 1, 129–169. Retrieved from https://www.centerforappreciativeinquiry.net/wp-content/uploads/2012/05/APPRECIATIVE_INQUIRY_IN_Orgnizational_life.pdf.

Covey, S. (1989). *The seven habits of highly successful people*. New York: Simon & Schuster.

Crabb, L. (1990). *Encouragement: The key to caring*. Grand Rapids, MI: Zondervan.

Csikszentmihalyi, M. (1997). *Finding flow: The psychology of engagement with everyday life*. New York: BasicBooks.

Darling-Hammond, L. (2010). *Education in a flat world: How our commitment to equity will shape the education of our future*. San Francisco, CA: Jossey-Bass.

Davidson, R., Weng, H. Y., Fox, A. S., Shackman, A. J., Stodola, D. E., Caldwell, J. Z. K., et al. (2013). Compassion training alters altruism and neural responses to suffer. *Psychological Science*, 24(7), 1171–1180.

Davidson, R., et al. (2003). Alterations in brain and immune function produced by mindfulness meditation. *Psychosomatic Medicine*, 65, 564–570.

Deci, E. L., Ryan, R. M., & Koestner, R. (1999). A meta-analytic review of experiments examining the effects of extrinsic rewards on instrisic motivation. *Psychological Bulletin*, 125(6), 627–668.

Diener, E. & Seligman, M. (2004). Beyond money. *Psychological Science in the Public Interest*, 5, 1–31.

Dweck, C. S. (2006). *Mindset: The new psychology of success*. New York: Ballantine Books.

Ferrari, B. T. (2012). *Power listening: Mastering the most critical business skill of all*. New York: Portfolio/Penguin.

Flook, L., Goldberg, S. B., Pinger, L., Bonus, K., & Davidson, R. J. (2013). Mindfulness for teachers: A pilot study to assess effects on stress, burnout, and teaching efficacy. *Mind, Brain, and Education*, 7, 182–195.

Flowers, S. & Stahl, B. (2011). *Living with your heart wide open: How mindfulness and compassion can free you from unworthiness, inadequacy and shame*. Oakland, CA: New Harbinger.

Frankl, V. (1984). *Man's search for meaning* (3rd ed.). Boston, MA: Beacon Press.

Fredrickson, B. L. (2013). *Love 2.0: How our supreme emotion affects everything we feel, think, do, and become*. New York: Penguin Books.

———. (2009). *Positivity*. New York: Crown.

———. (2008). Promoting positive affect. In M. Eid & R. Larsen (Eds.), *The science of subjective wellbeing*, pp. 449–468. New York: Guildford Press.

———. (2004). The broaden-and-build theory of positive emotions. *Philosophical Transactions of the Royal Society of London B: Biological Sciences*, 359(1449), 1367–1378. doi:10.1098/rstb.2004.1512.

Fredrickson, B. L. & Losada, M. F. (2005). Positive affect and the complex dynamics of human flourishing. *American Psychologist*, 60, 678–686.

Greenberg, M. T., Weissberg, R. P., Utne O'Brien, M., Zins, J. E., Fredericks, L., & Resnik, H. (2003). Enhancing school-based prevention and youth development through coordinated social, emotional, and academic-learning. *American Psychologist, 58,* 451–466.

Greene, M. (1978). *Landscapes of learning.* New York: Teachers College Press.

Gordon, M. (2011). Listening as embracing the other: Martin Buber's philosophy of dialogue. *Educational Theory, 61,* 207–219. doi:10.1111/j.1741-5446.2011.00400.x.

Graham, C. (2009). *Happiness around the world: The paradox of happy peasants and miserable millionaires.* Oxford: Oxford University Press.

Haidt, J. (2006). *The happiness hypothesis: Finding modern truth in ancient wisdom.* New York: Basic Books.

Hanson, K. (2017). *A Mindful teaching community: Possibilities for teacher professional learning.* Lanham, MD: Lexington Books.

Harris, R. (2009). *ACT made simple: An easy-to-read primer on acceptance and committment therapy.* Oakland, CA: New Harbinger Publications.

Hart, T. N. (1980). *The art of Christian living.* New York/Mahwah, NJ: Paulist Press.

Haybron, D. (2008). Happiness, the self and human flourishing. *Utilitas, 20,* 21–49.

Higgins, C. (2011). *The good life of teaching: An ethics of professional practice.* Malden, MA: Wiley-Blackwell.

Hoban, G. (2010). *Teacher learning for educational change.* New York: McGraw Hill.

Hodges, T. D. & Asplund, J. (2010). Strengths development in the workplace. In P. A. Linley, S. Harrington, & N. Garcea (Eds.), *The Oxford handbook of positive psychology,* pp. 213–221. New York: Oxford University Press.

Houston, J. M. (1996). *In pursuit of happiness: Finding genuine fulfillment in life.* Vancouver: Regent College Publishing.

Inoue, N. (2015). *Beyond actions: Psychology of action research for mindful educational improvement.* New York, New York: Peter Lang.

———. (2012). *Mirrors of the mind: Introduction to mindful ways of thinking education.* New York: Peter Lang.

Kabat-Zinn, J. (1994). *Wherever you go, there you are.* New York: Hyperion.

———. (2003). Mindfulness-based interventions in context. *Clinical Psychology: Science and Practice,* 10(2), 144–156.

Kesebir, J. & Diener, E. (2008). In pursuit of happiness: Empirical answers to philosophical questions. *Perspectives on Psychological Science,* 3(2), 117–125.

Kreeft, P. (1990). *Making choices: Practical wisdom for everday moral decisions.* Ann Arbor, MI: Servant Publications.

Jennings, P. A., Frank, J. L., Snowberg, K. E., Coccia, M. A., & Greenberg, M. T. (2013). Improving classroom learning environments by cultivating awareness and resilience in education (CARE): Results of a randomized-controlled trial. *School Psychology Quarterly,* 28, 374–390.

Jennings, P. A. & Greenberg, M. (2009). The pro-social classroom: Teacher social and emotional competence in relation to student and classroom outcomes. *Review of Educational Research* 79, 491–525.

Jones, S. M. (2011). Supportive listening. *International Journal of Listening,* 25, 851–863.

Langer, E. (2005). *On becoming an artist: Reinventing yourself through mindful creativity.* New York: Ballantine Books.

———. (1997). *The power of mindful learning.* Reading, MA: Addison-Wesley.

———. (1993). A mindful education. *Educational Psychologist,* 28, 43–50.

———. (1989). *Mindfulness.* USA: Da Capo Books/Perseus Group.

Layard, R. (2005). *Happiness: Lessons from a new science.* New York: Penguin Books.

Leana, C., Appelbaum, E., & Shevchuk, I. (2009). Work process and quality of care in early childhood education: The role of job crafting. *Academy of Management Journal,* 52, 1169–1192.

Levinson, M. (2015). Moral injury and the ethics of educational injustice. *Harvard Educational Review,* 85(2), 203–228.

Lutz, A., Brefczynski-Lewis, J., Johnstone, T., & Davidson, R. J. (2008). Regulation of the neural circuitry of emotion by compassion meditation: Effects of meditative expertise. *PloS ONE*, 3. doi: 10.1371/journal.pone.0001897.

Lyubomirsky, S. (2007). *The how of happiness: A scientific approach to getting the life you want*. New York: Penguin Books.

MacDonald, E. & Shirley, D. (2009). *The mindful teacher*. New York: Teachers College Press.

Marks, N. (2011). *The happiness manifesto*. (TED eBook).

Martin A. J. & Marsh, H. W. (2006). Academic resilience and its psychological and educational correlates: A construct validity approach. *Psychology in Schools*, 43, 267–281.

Marturano, J. (2014). *Finding the space to lead: A practical guide to mindful leadership*. New York: Bloomsbury Press.

Meiklejohn, J., Philips, C., Freedman, M. E., Griffin, M. L., Biegel, G., Roach, A., Frank, J., Burke, C., Pinger, L., Soloway, G., Isberg, R., Sibinga, E., Grossman, L., & Saltzman, A. (2012). Integrating mindfulness training into K–12 education: Fostering the resilience of teachers and students. *Mindfulness*, 3, 291–307.

Merriam-Webster Online Dictionary. Retrieved September 11, 2015.

Milton, Mark. (2000). Listening is everybody's business: Campaign for the promotion of listening: "To lend an ear is to lend a hand": A column of Befrienders International. *Crisis: The Journal of Crisis Intervention and Suicide Prevention*, 21, 52–54.

Mineyama, S., Tsutsumi, A., Takao, S., Nishiuchi, K., & Kawakami, N. (2007). Supervisors' attitudes and skills for active listening with regard to working conditions and psychological stress reactions among subordinates. *Journal of Occupational Health*, 49, 81–87.

Nakamura, J. & Csikszentmihalyi, M. (2014). The concept of flow. In *Flow and the foundations of positive psychology*, pp. 239–263. Springer Netherlands.

Neff, K. (2003). Self-compassion: An alternative conceptualization of a healthy attitude toward oneself. *Self and Identity*, 2, 85–101.

———. (2009a). Self-compassion. In M. Leary & H. Hoyle (Eds.), *Handbook of individual differences in social behavior*, pp. 561–573. New York: Gilford Press.

———. (2009b). The role of self-compassion development: A healthier way to relate to one-self. *Human Development*, 52, 211–214.

Newmark, R., Krahnke, K., & Seaton, L. (2013). Incorporating mindfulness mediation In the classroom. *Journal of the Academy of Business & Economics*, 13, 79–95.

Noble, T. & McGrath, H. (2008). The positive educational practices framework: A tool for facilitating the work of educational psychologists in promoting pupil wellbeing. *Educational and Child Psychology*, 25(2), 119–134.

Nussbaum, M. (1996). *The therapy of desire*. Princeton, NJ: Princeton University Press.

———. (2011). *Creating capabilities: The human development approach*. Cambridge: The Belknap Press of Harvard University Press.

Online Etymology Dictionary. Retrieved September 11, 2015.

Palmer, P. J. (1998). *Courage to teach*. San Francisco, CA: Jossey-Bass.

———. (1999a). Evoking the spirit in public education. *Educational leadership*, 56, 6–11.

———. (1999b). *Let your life speak: Listening for the voice of vocation*. San Francisco, CA: Jossey-Bass.

———. (2004). *A hidden wholeness: The journey toward an undivided life*. San Francisco, CA: Jossey-Bass.

Park, N., Peterson, C., & Seligman, M. E. (2004). Strengths of character and well-being. *Journal of Social and Clinical Psychology*, 23, 603–619.

Pasupathi, M. & Billitteri, J. (2015). Being and becoming through being heard: Listener effects on stories and selves. *International Journal of Listening*, 29, 67–84.

Pattakos, A. (2010). *Prisoners of our thoughts: Viktor Frankl's principles for discovering meaning in life and work* (2nd ed.). San Francisco, CA: Berrett-Koehler.

Pattersen, K., Grenny, J., McMillan, R., & Switzler, A. (2002). *Crucial conversations: Tools for talking when stakes are high*. New York: McGraw Hill.

Pence, M. E. & James, T. A. (2015). The role of sex differences in the examination of personality and active-empathic listening: An initial exploration. *International Journal of Listening*, 29, 85–94.

Petersen, J. (2007). *Why don't we listen better?* Portland, OR: Petersen Publications.

Quinn, R. & Carl, N. M. (2015). Teacher activist organizations and the development of professional agency. *Teachers and Teaching: Theory and Practice*, 21(6), 745–758.

Ragoonaden, K. (2015). Mindful education and wellbeing. In K. Ragoonaden (Ed.), *Mindful teaching and learning: Developing a pedagogy of wellbeing*, pp. 172–179. Lanham, MD: Lexington Books.

Ragoonaden, K. & Bullock, S. (2016). *Mindfulness and critical friendship*. Lanham, MD: Lexington.

Rassmussen, D. (1999). Human flourishing and the appeal to human nature. *Social Philosophy and Policy*, 16(1), 1–43.

Rath, T. (2006). *Vital friends: The people you can't afford to live without*. New York: Simon and Schuster.

Rath, T. & Harter, J. K. (2010). *Wellbeing: The five essential elements*. New York: Simon and Schuster.

Rechtschaffen, D. J. (2014). *The way of mindful education: Cultivating wellbeing in teachers and students*. New York: W. W. Norton & Company.

Rodgers, C. & Raider-Roth, M. (2006). Presence in teaching. *Teachers and Teaching*, 12(3), 2652–2687.

Roeser, R. W., Skinner, E., Beers, J., & Jennings, P. A. (2012). Mindfulness training and teachers' professional development: An emerging area of research and practice. *Child Development Perspectives*, 6, 167–173.

Sackney, L. & Walker, K. (2007). Sustainable innovation in exemplary schools. *International Journal of Interdisciplinary Social Sciences*, 1, 1–10.

Samaras, A. (2011). *Self-study teacher research: Improving your practice through collaborative inquiry*. Thousand Oaks, CA: Sage.

Scharmer, O. (2009). *Theory U: Learning from the future as it emerges*. San Francisco, CA: Berrett-Koehler Publishing.

Scharmer, O. & Kaufer, K. (2013). *Leading from the emerging future: From ego-system to eco-system economies*. San Francisco, CA: Berrett-Koehler Publishers, Inc.

Schonert-Reichl, K. & Lawlor, M. (2010). The effects of a mindfulness-based education program on pre- and early adolescents' wellbeing and social and emotional competence. *Mindfulness*, 1(3), 137–151.

Seigel, D. (2007). *The mindful brain: Reflection and attunement in the cultivation of wellbeing*. New York: Norton.

Seligman, M. (2009). Positive education: Positive psychology and classroom interventions. *Oxford Review of Education*, 35(3), 293–311.

———. (2011). *Flourish: A visionary new understanding of happiness and wellbeing*. New York: Free Press.

Sen, A. (2009). *The idea of justice*. London: Allen Lane.

Sergiovanni, T. J. (1994). Organizations or communities? Changing the metaphor changes the theory. *Educational Administration Quarterly*, 30(2), 214–220.

Sergiovanni, T. J. & Starratt, R. J. (1993). *Supervision: A redefinition*. New York: McGraw-Hill Education.

Shipley, S. D. (2010). Listening: A concept analysis. *Nursing Forum*, 45(2), 125–134.

Spitzer, R. (2000). *Healing the culture: A commonsense philosophy of happiness, freedom and the life issues*. San Francisco: Ignatius Press.

Starratt, R. J. (2004). Leadership of the contested terrain of education for democracy. *Journal of Educational Administration*, 42(6), 724–731.

Thich Nhat Hanh (n.d.). Thich Nhat Hanh's tea meditation. Retrieved from http://www.oprah.com/own-super-soul-sunday/thich-nhat-hanhs-tea-meditation-video.

Vanier, J. (2001). *Made for happiness: Discovering the meaning of life with Aristotle*. (K. Spink, Trans.). New York: House of Anansi Press, Ltd.

Weger, H. Jr., Castle, G., & Emmett, M. C. (2010). Active listening in peer interviews: The influence of message paraphrasing on perceptions of listening skill. *International Journal of Listening*, 24(1), 34–49.

Wheatley, M. J. (1999). When complex systems fail: New roles for leaders. *Leader to Leader*, 11, 28–34. doi:10.1002/ltl.40619991108.

———. (2005). *Finding our way: Leadership for an uncertain time*. San Francisco, CA: Berrett-Koehler.

Whitney, D. & Trosten-Bloom, A. (2010). *The power of appreciative inquiry: A practical guide to positive change*. (2nd ed.). San Francisco: CA: Berrett-Koehler.

Worline, M. & Dutton, J. E. (2017). *Awakening compassion at work: The quiet power that elevates people and organizations*. San Franciscio, CA: Berrett-Koehler Publishers.

Wrzesniewski, A. & Dutton, J. E. (2001). Crafting a job: Revisioning employees as active crafters of their work. *The Academy of Management Review*, 26(2), 179–201.

Young, C. K., Kashdan, T. B., & Macatee, R. (2014). Strength balance and implicit strength measurement: New considerations for research on strengths of character. *The Journal of Positive Psychology*.

Zeichner, K. (2010). Rethinking the connections between campus courses and field experiences in college- and university-based teacher education. *Journal of Teacher Education*, 61(1–2), 81–99.

Zins, J., Weissberg, R., Wang, M., & Walberg, H. J. (Eds.). (2004). *Building academic success on social and emotional learning: What does the research say?* New York: Teachers College Press.

Index

About the Authors

Dr. Sabre Cherkowski, PhD, is an associate professor and director of the Centre for Mindful Engagement in the Faculty of Education at the University of British Columbia. She teaches and researches in the areas of organizational wellbeing; leadership in learning communities; professional learning; collaboration; diversity and education; and teacher education. She brings her experiences as a teacher, coach, and parent to her passion for exploring flourishing in educational contexts.

Kelly Hanson is a doctoral student at the University of British Columbia, Canada. For the past twelve years, she has been a public middle school teacher in British Columbia and Ontario. She is a faculty advisor in the newly designed INSPIRE Bachelor of Education program at University of British Columbia, Okanagan. Her research interests include the intersections between teacher education, mindfulness, and the field of curriculum studies, and the possibilities of mindfulness to enliven autobiographical/relational understanding in the lives of educators and students to create more wellbeing in teaching and learning. In 2014, Kelly co-founded 4C Consulting to support other educators to develop mindful practices with the intention of contributing to self/community thriving

Dr. Keith Walker enjoys a joint appointment in the Department of Educational Administration at the University of Saskatchewan. His recognized areas of work include educational governance and policy-making, leadership philosophies and practices, community and interpersonal relations, organizational development and capacity-building, and applied and professional ethics. He brings over thirty-five years of experience as a manager, teacher, minister, leader, scholar, and educational administrator in public and social sectors. His formal education has been in the disciplines of physical education, sports administration, theology, education, educational administration, and philosophy.

www.ingramcontent.com/pod-product-compliance
Lightning Source LLC
Chambersburg PA
CBHW021821270326
41932CB00007B/286